Milady's
Situational Problems
for the
Cosmetology Student

Milady's Situational Problems for the Cosmetology Student

Catherine M. Frangie

THOMSON

DELMAR LEARNING

Milady's Situational Problems for the Cosmetology Student
Catherine Frangie

President,
 Milady
Dawn Gerrain

Director of
 Editorial:
Sherry Gomoll

Acquisitions Editor:
Stephen Smith

Editorial Assistant:
Courtney VanAuskas

Director of
 Production:
Wendy A. Troeger

Production
 Coordinator:
Nina Tucciarelli

Composition:
TypeShoppe II

Marketing Specialist:
Sandra Bruce

Marketing Assistant
Kasmira Koniszewski

Library of Congress Cataloging-in-Publication Card Number:
2002074216
ISBN 978-1-40183-895-2
ISBN 1-40183-895-2

NOTICE TO THE READER

Contents

INTRODUCTION

Welcome to the professional beauty industry! You have chosen to pursue a wonderful and exciting career opportunity. It takes honing many skills and developing many characteristics to be successful in the beauty industry, but perhaps the most important skill is the ability to think through the situation at hand, then choose the best, most equitable solution for all the parties involved. Remember, you will be working with lots of different people—clients, coworkers, managers, vendors—and each will have his or her own perception and perspective on every encounter and every situation. While there will be many, many possible outcomes to every experience and encounter, as a professional cosmetologist you will need to concentrate on fostering positive experiences for yourself and your clients to make a living.

Milady's Situational Problems for the Cosmetology Student was created to help acquaint you with the types of situations and dilemmas you will encounter in your daily life as a professional cosmetologist, and to give you an opportunity to sharpen your decision-making and relationship skills. As you read the stories in the book and then prepare to answer the questions that follow each story, keep in mind that this workbook gives you an opportunity now to determine how you will handle similar situations later in your professional career. So take your time, think each situation through, and make the best decision you can, based on the information you are given.

Once again, I want to congratulate you on your professional choice and wish you the best of luck in your career!

—Catherine M. Frangie

PREFACE

How to Use This Book

Milady's Situational Problems for the Cosmetology Student was created for use with *Milady's Standard Cosmetology*, 2004 edition. *Milady's Situational Problems for the Cosmetology Student* was written to correspond to the core textbook by providing students with real-life scenarios that illustrate core concepts and points.

This book is organized by chapter, corresponding with the chapters in the core textbook, and each scenario is categorized by topic, making it easy for students to look up information in the text. As students work their way through the scenarios, they will have an opportunity to build on their working knowledge of the principles and theories taught in *Milady's Standard Cosmetology*, and see how these theories apply to everyday salon life.

There are many ways that this book can be used in conjunction with the core textbook: after the completion of reading assignments, as homework assignments, during theory class, to review for tests, or in preparation for clinic work. Regardless of how the book is used in the classroom, it is recommended that these scenarios be used as a basis for further student discussions and debate.

Part I—ORIENTATION

Chapter 2

Life Skills

THE PSYCHOLOGY OF SUCCESS

John always dreamed of becoming a successful professional. He has taken a position with a prestigious salon where he has been working for five years. John drives an expensive automobile and rents a pricey apartment in a chic neighborhood. His wardrobe consists of designer and name-brand clothing, fashionable shoes and accessories, and John is always impeccably dressed. John spends a lot of time and money on his appearance and he wishes he was better compensated for his work because he has difficulty paying his other expenses—his car and rent— each month, but he is reluctant to reduce his expenses because he is concerned that the salon's well-to-do clients won't patronize him if he doesn't live up to their standard of living. Because he works about 70 hours per week, he doesn't have a lot of time to devote to other activities. John hardly ever sees his friends and family, and rarely takes any time to enjoy sports or music, his favorite pastimes.

1. John's self-esteem appears to be based on:
   A. his inner strengths
   B. his ability to possess things
   C. his ability to care for his things
   D. his physical strengths

2. John has used the technique of visualization to:
   A. picture himself as a complete success
   B. improve his sleep
   C. picture himself as a complete hair stylist
   D. improve his ability to concentrate

3. A truly successful person does not:
   A. get enough rest
   B. pace himself to prevent fatigue
   C. allow business to be the only focus of his life
   D. socialize with people outside of his business

4. John's lifestyle requires him to spend all of his time:
   A. visiting with family
   B. exercising
   C. visiting with friends
   D. working

5. John's definition of success includes:
   A. dividing his time between work and pleasure
   B. increasing his education
   C. having a daily exercise routine
   D. keeping up appearances

6. Whose definition of success is John attempting to achieve?
   A. His family's
   B. His coworker's
   C. His client's
   D. His friend's

TIME MANAGEMENT

Ramona is a busy person. She has a part-time job, a small child, attends school, and has many other tasks and responsibilities to attend to each day. Now that she is about to graduate from beauty school and begin to look for a job in a salon, Ramona knows that she has to become better organized, but she always feels frustrated by how much she has to do and how little time she has to do it in. Ramona has good intentions but often gets so caught up in the day's activities and events that she forgets important errands she needs to run or appointments she has made. Ramona has resolved to utilize her time more efficiently.

7. The first thing Ramona must do is:
   A. reorganize her living room to make the flow of furniture work better
   B. prioritize the list of tasks that need to be done in the order of most to least important
   C. take on an additional project for her current employer
   D. drop every other task she has until she finds a salon job

8. Ramona needs to have some specific time with her young child each day. She can accomplish this by:
   A. taking the child to school an hour later each day
   B. designing a schedule for herself that includes blocks of unstructured time
   C. taking her child to work with her each evening
   D. designing a play space in the salon

9. Which of the following will NOT save Ramona time in her busy schedule?
   A. Reducing as much stress as possible
   B. Saying "no" when being asked to take on more than she can handle
   C. Relying on others to problem-solve and uncover solutions she can use
   D. Taking a time-out whenever she is frustrated, overwhelmed, irritated, worried, or feeling guilty

10. When Ramona is feeling overwhelmed by the circumtances of her hectic life, she could try a technique called:
    A. shallow breathing
    B. deep breathing
    C. shallow sighing
    D. deep sighing

11. To aid Ramona in remembering important notes and reminders, she should carry:
    A. a memo pad or day planner
    B. her favorite music CD
    C. a computer
    D. her address book

12. Ramona might consider scheduling her time in ____ intervals to study for a major exam.
    A. 10-minute
    B. 15-minute
    C. 30-minute
    D. 60-minute

13. To make the most of her time, Ramona should schedule activities that require alert, clear thinking during times when she is:
    A. wearing comfortable clothing
    B. distracted and can't concentrate
    C. highly energetic and able to focus
    D. not feeling well and needing medication

14. Which of the following is NOT a healthy way for Ramona to reward herself for a job well done?
    A. Taking a bubble bath
    B. Going to a movie
    C. Taking a nap
    D. Smoking a cigarette

15. Another activity Ramona must consider scheduling to promote clear thinking and planning is:
    A. exercising
    B. eating dessert
    C. reading magazines
    D. oversleeping

16. Which of the following tools would help Ramona the most to keep herself focused on the tasks she needs to complete each day?
    A. A mission statement
    B. A goal statement
    C. A to-do list
    D. A long-range plan

STUDY SKILLS

Hector is a dedicated student who wants to progress through school and become a licensed professional. While he is happy to be in school, he has difficulty staying focused during lectures, and studying for and taking exams. He usually ends up cramming the night before an exam, even for important tests that cover many topics. Hector is frustrated and wants to have an easier time of this facet of his schooling. He knows that he is a capable and serious student, and he is willing try some new techniques to lessen his fears and anxiety about test-taking.

17. What is missing from Hector's educational background?
    A. A desire to work hard
    B. Good study skills
    C. A desire to succeed
    D. Good people skills

18. When Hector feels overwhelmed by his courses and upcoming tests, he can focus on ___ to feel better about himself and his progress.
    A. rereading the entire chapter in his textbook
    B. checking out more reference books from the school library
    C. accomplishing small tasks, one at a time
    D. other activities that make him feel more confident

19. Instead of cramming the night before an exam, Hector should:
    A. study for up to three hours at a stretch two days before the exam
    B. study for one hour just before taking the exam
    C. study in small intervals when the lesson is presented and it won't be necessary to review before the test
    D. study the day's lessons each day, then review all the material before the exam

20. Which of the following techniques will help Hector stay focused when his mind begins to wander in class?
    A. Write notes to fellow students
    B. Think about becoming a successful professional
    C. Write down key words and discuss them with the instructor
    D. Look up definitions of terms in his textbook

21. If Hector decides to form and/or join a study group, what should he look for in the group?
    A. Students who will give him the information he needs
    B. Students who are willing to be helpful and supportive
    C. Students who have the same interests he has
    D. Students who have a good sense of humor and are fun to be with

22. If Hector was to find a "study buddy," what would that person's job be?
    A. To introduce him to other students
    B. To eat lunch with him
    C. To help him stay focused on studying
    D. To practice finger waving with

LEARNING STYLES

Mrs. Jones teaches several cosmetology classes each day. In her early morning lecture, there are four students who sit in the front row. One student is Janice who diligently reads the assigned sections in the textbook and has an excellent memory for facts and details. Another student, Delores, prefers it when Mrs. Jones demonstrates techniques, and she is always willing to be the first student to try the new technique herself once it has been discussed and explained to the class. The third student, James, is an active observer in every class and he likes to talk about what he is learning with his classmates. And Jill, the fourth student, is always asking Mrs. Jones how what she is describing would relate to a real-life salon situation.

23. What type of learner is Janice?
    A. Interactive learner
    B. Reader/listener learner
    C. Systematic learner
    D. Intuitive learner

24. What type of learner is Delores?
    A. Interactive learner
    B. Reader/listener learner
    C. Systematic learner
    D. Intuitive learner

25. What type of learner is James?
    A. Interactive learner
    B. Reader/listener learner
    C. Systematic learner
    D. Intuitive learner

26. What type of learner is Jill?
    A. Interactive learner
    B. Reader/listener learner
    C. Systematic learner
    D. Intuitive learner

27. A reader/listener learner is someone who asks the question:
    A. who
    B. what
    C. where
    D. why

28. Intuitive learners like to learn through:
    A. trial and error
    B. reading and writing
    C. memorizing and reciting
    D. watching and observing

29. Interactive learners most appreciate instructors who are:
    A. detailed and formal
    B. aloof and cool
    C. sympathetic and friendly
    D. blunt and direct

30. Systematic learners study best:
    A. with one other person
    B. in a study group
    C. by themselves
    D. over the telephone

ETHICS

Hakim and Jake are senior stylists and assistant managers at the Bella Luna Salon and Spa. Both have excellent technical skills and both are attractive-looking professionals who are intelligent and capable. Hakim's behavior is hallmarked by a sense of calm: he manages his fellow coworkers with honest and open communications, he is respectful of clients, and he never gossips. However, when he has problems at home, he often calls in sick for the day with little notice to the salon. Jake, the other senior stylist, is quick to complain about other people, is sometimes bossy and uncaring about the feelings of others, and he acts as if the salon's rules and policies do not pertain to him. But Jake is always at work, on time, and he rarely ever takes unscheduled time off from work. Adam, the salon's owner, has a salon manager's job opening to fill, and Hakim and Jake are the two candidates from whom he must choose.

31. In making his decision, Adam must choose the person who is best at:
    A. fixing haircolor mistakes
    B. socializing with other stylists
    C. honestly speaking to stylists
    D. appointment scheduling

32. In assessing Hakim and Jake, which of the following does NOT indicate a high standard of professionalism?
    A. Identifying one's values
    B. Avoiding all conflict
    C. Maintaining one's principles
    D. Developing a sense of genuine concern for others

33. Which of the following is NOT an ethical characteristic for Hakim and Jake to aspire to?
    A. Compassion
    B. Attentiveness
    C. Punctuality
    D. Uncooperativeness

34. Based on Jake's behavior, what type of personality traits is he likely displaying when he is asked to manage the salon?
    A. A pleasant, agreeable personality
    B. A difficult, disagreeable personality
    C. A calm, gentle personality
    D. A difficult but joking personality

35. As a caregiver, Hakim must be able to practice:
    A. self-sufficiency
    B. self-care
    C. self-indulgence
    D. self-deprivation

36. When determining Jake and Hakim's sense of integrity, Adam will need to assess:
    A. if their communications and actions match their personalities
    B. if their behaviors and actions match their values
    C. if their values and sense of humor match their behavior
    D. if their behaviors and actions match their personalities

37. For Jake to display a good sense of integrity, he would have to behave in the following manner:
    A. use high-end products only
    B. provide the best scalp massage in the salon
    C. market to clients from previous employers
    D. recommend products and services from which the client can benefit

38. When Jake gossips with other stylists about a client's personal situation, he is lacking:
    A. deception
    B. personality
    C. discretion
    D. politeness

39. Which of the following characteristics indicates that Hakim is extending ethical behavior to his communication with customers and the other people with whom he works?
    A. Buying lunch
    B. Being indirect
    C. Being direct
    D. Wearing trendy clothing

PERSONALITY DEVELOPMENT AND ATTITUDE

Marcia is the receptionist at the Salon Omega. One of her most important duties is to schedule clients effectively and efficiently so that neither the stylists nor clients are waiting for long periods of time. Marcia has scheduled Mr. Hatch for a haircut and scalp massage with Jane for 6 P.M. It is almost 6:20 P.M. when he calls from his cell phone to say that he is stuck in traffic and would like to change his appointment to 7 P.M. In front of Marcia are Jane's 7 P.M. and 7:30 P.M. appointments, so there is no way she can reschedule Mr. Hatch for this evening. Marcia, annoyed at him, says, "Well, if you had called immediately, I might have been able to move a later appointment up. You should have called sooner to reschedule, like when you first got stuck in the traffic jam! There's nothing I can do now. Jane has no openings until next week." Mr. Hatch explains, "I thought the traffic would clear up sooner and that I'd make it in time. I'm sorry if I caused any problems. I'd like to make another appointment." Marcia tells him, "Well, you have caused problems. Jane is sitting here waiting for you while two other clients are already here and she could have been servicing them!" Marcia looks at the appointment calendar and says that she can make an appointment for him for the following week. But, she warns, "You have to be sure you're going to make it in time and if you can't be on time, you have to call me right away and not leave us hanging here." Mr. Hatch said he would like to take the appointment. Marcia marks his name in the calendar and then completes the call.

40. From her response, what kind of attitude does Marcia have about people who are late?
    A. She is understanding and helpful
    B. She is sad and tearful
    C. She is impatient and distrusting
    D. She is angry and abusive

41. How would you rate Marcia's ability to handle the situation with Mr. Hatch tactfully?
     A. Excellent—she was able to reschedule Mr. Hatch's appointment without incident
     B. Good—she clearly stated that his tardiness could not happen again
     C. Fair—she wasn't very sympathetic but managed to reschedule the client
     D. Poor—she argued with the client and he promised never to return to the salon

42. How should Marcia have handled the conversation with Mr. Hatch?
     A. She should have became annoyed and repeated that his tardiness was a problem
     B. She should have flown into a rage at his inconsiderate behavior
     C. She should have yelled into the phone that Jane didn't want to service clients like him
     D. She should have let him know that missing his appointment was a problem, and asked him if he'd prefer to be the last client of the day to give him ample time to get to the salon

43. How sensitive was Marcia to Mr. Hatch?
     A. Extremely
     B. Moderately
     C. Somewhat
     D. Not sensitive at all

44. Based on Marcia's response to this situation, what do think her values and goals are?
     A. Empathy and harmony
     B. Sensitivity and caring
     C. Precision and efficiency
     D. Accusation and blame

45. What will likely be the effect of Marcia's comments on Mr. Hatch?
    A. He will feel understood
    B. He will feel reprimanded
    C. He will feel insignificant
    D. He will feel guilty

HUMAN RELATIONS

Tyrone is a distributor sales consultant who is calling on Eva, a salon owner, whose two-week-old order has still not been delivered. Eva is angry because she has missed several opportunities to make retail sales and to service clients because she can't get the products she needs, and she complains about this to Tyrone. Frustrated because Eva is the fourth salon owner he has called on this week with the same complaint, Tyrone slams his sales book shut and tells Eva, "I've told you already that the products are back-ordered from the manufacturer and there's nothing I can do about it. If you aren't interested in seeing this new brush line, then I guess there's nothing else I can do for you!"

46. Tyrone's reaction to Eva indicated that he was:
    A. aware of the problems with the delivery and had an alternative plan
    B. not rattled by her complaints and able to offer another solution
    C. unprepared for her complaints and took them personally
    D. aware that she was overreacting out of frustration and displayed a lack of communication

47. If Tyrone had a strong sense of his abilities, how would he have behaved with Eva?
    A. Just as he did
    B. He would have patted her hand and told her whatever he could to calm her down
    C. He would have blamed his manager and had Eva call him right away
    D. He would call her with a delivery date and propose some alternative options

48. Had Tyrone really been listening to Eva's complaint, what opportunity might he have been presented with?
    A. The chance to sell her a new product line to try
    B. The chance to take an additional order
    C. The chance to transfer her account to another representative
    D. The chance to tell off his manager and feel justified in doing so

49. What would have been the best way for Tyrone to attend to Eva's needs?
    A. Ignore her complaints and move on with his sales call
    B. Join her in complaining about the company
    C. Agree with her complaint and ask what he could do to help her in the short term
    D. Simply listen to her and offer no reaction at all

50. From Tyrone's reaction to Eva, what can you infer about his job satisfaction?
    A. He is very happy at work and looking forward to being promoted
    B. He is frustrated by his working conditions and is able to discuss this with his manager
    C. He is happy at work and looks forward to his next paycheck
    D. He is unhappy at work and is not handling his frustrations in a positive manner

Chapter 3

YOUR PROFESSIONAL IMAGE

BEAUTY AND WELLNESS

Marcella is always rushed and is frequently late for work. To save time in the morning, she sometimes showers in the evening before going to bed so that the time she spends getting ready for work in the morning is less. Marcella awakens a half hour before she needs to leave her house, quickly washes her face, brushes her teeth, puts on her makeup, dresses, and flies out the door to get to the salon. On several days, after working at the salon, she goes to her evening job, often without freshening her clothes, herself, or her makeup. Her clients and colleagues noticeably pull away from her when she is speaking to them or in close contact with them. Behind her back, some of Marcella's colleagues make fun of her and call her names like "sloppy" and "disheveled" because she is always late, seemingly forgetful, and never looks well put together or freshly bathed. Marcella is always tired and she is becoming increasingly unhappy.

51. Does it sound like Marcella is enjoying good health?
    A. Yes, she is able to go to work every day and earn a living
    B. Yes, her mind, body, and spirit seem to be working cooperatively
    C. No, she is busy but able to maintain two jobs
    D. No, her mind, body, and spirit do not seem to be working cooperatively

52. One of the most important things that Marcella seems to be lacking is:
    A. balance
    B. money
    C. commitment
    D. education

53. Based on the reaction from Marcella's colleagues, how would you rate her personal hygiene?
    A. Excellent
    B. Very good
    C. Good
    D. Fair

54. Which of the following should Marcella NOT do to improve her personal hygiene between jobs?
    A. Brush her teeth
    B. Use underarm deodorant
    C. Freshen her makeup
    D. Douse herself with perfume

55. What is most likely the cause of coworkers and clients pulling away from her when Marcella is speaking to them?
    A. Fresh breath
    B. Foul language
    C. Bad breath
    D. Complicated language

56. What does Marcella's disheveled appearance say about her professionalism?
    A. That she is a meticulous professional
    B. That she is proud to be in her profession
    C. That she is happy with her job and lifestyle
    D. That she is feeling stress and cannot manage her time

Paige is in her early twenties and she loves to wear her hair with styling glue. She describes her style as the "dirty grunge look." She often wears the sleeves of her shirt rolled up high so her tattoos can be seen. Paige loves to wear dark, colorful makeup applied in an avant-garde fashion. Since she really needs a job, she has decided to apply at the luxury spa that has just opened a few blocks from her home. A couple of days before her interview, Paige goes into the spa and observes that the spa employees are all wearing simple black clothing with white smocks over them. She notices that their hair is styled into simple and classic looks, and their makeup is simple, employing natural colors and techniques. Paige decides that in order to have a shot at the job she wants so desperately, she will dress in accordance with the other spa staffers during her interview and then later, slip into her own style once she has gotten the job.

57. How should Paige go about finding the best place to work?
    A. Visit several salons and determine which one is most in line with her own sense of style
    B. Apply for a position at a mall salon and take the job when it is offered
    C. Agree to be a salon assistant for at least one year before she decides
    D. Ask her friends what type of salon they are looking for and follow their lead

58. What is the energy and image of the spa Paige is interviewing at?
    A. A chic spa with celebrity clients
    B. A low-cost salon that specializes in short layered cuts
    C. A high-end spa that has an exclusive clientele
    D. A high-end color-only salon

59. What type of salon seems most appropriate for someone with Paige's sense of style to work in?
    A. A color-only salon catering to clients who want to cover gray hair
    B. A moderately priced salon that caters to young clients who have a sense of adventure
    C. A moderately priced salon that caters to business people
    D. A mall salon that caters to families and children

60. Is Paige's approach to getting this job ethical?
    A. Yes, because she really needs the job and she will be a good employee
    B. Yes, because they should be hiring her for her skill and not her appearance
    C. No, because she isn't being honest about who she really is
    D. No, because she can help them change the salon's culture

Peter loves to have a good time, and almost every day after working at the salon, he meets up with his buddies to hang out. They often go to one another's apartment and order pizza, drinks, and watch television until late into the night. Often, because Peter is so tired, he sleeps on his friend's couch, then gets up the next day and goes directly to work. His salon coworkers always know when Peter has been out with his friends the night before because he is often barely awake, unshaven, and wearing the same clothes he wore the day before. Peter gets teased by the other salon employees for being a "free spirit," but Allie, the salon manager, isn't as able to let his messy appearance go because after one of these evenings, he is often so disheveled that he is off-putting to salon clients. Allie decides to have a conversation with Peter about his appearance and general hygiene.

61. The best time for Allie to approach Peter would be:
    A. when they are in a staff meeting
    B. when Peter is with a client
    C. when they are alone in the salon
    D. when Allie is in a managers meeting

62. What should Allie discuss with Peter?
    A. His personal appearance and its affect on the salon's clients
    B. His attitude about partying too much
    C. His irresponsible behavior toward his family
    D. His favorite television shows

63. What could Peter do to make sure he is fresh for work, even on nights when he doesn't sleep at home?
    A. Take a shower the evening before so he doesn't have to worry about it in the morning
    B. Spray himself with some cologne on the way in to work
    C. Keep clean clothing in his car and freshen up before arriving at the salon
    D. Spray his worn clothing with something that eliminates odors

64. The image that Peter is projecting to clients suggests that he is:
    A. a serious professional concerned with learning more on the job
    B. between apartments and sleeping wherever he can
    C. concerned with doing an excellent job at the salon
    D. sad and unhappy in his work

HEALTHY MIND AND BODY

Carol's day begins early with getting her two small children off to school and making sure she is on time for work. She is the salon manager at a very busy mall salon in the center of town. The salon is open daily from 9 A.M. to 9 P.M. and Carol has 13 employees to manage. In addition to her work situation, Carol is going through a divorce from her husband of 10 years, and she is often very sad and angry about what their relationship has disintegrated into. And because of the divorce, money is very tight. Lately, Carol finds herself snapping at her children and their baby-sitter when they do not act according to the schedule she has set or when they make demands that she feels are too much for her to handle. Last week, she had a very unpleasant conversation with the salon's owners who accused her of having a bad attitude after a couple of the stylists called them to complain about Carol. Carol is tired and frustrated, and she feels trapped in a routine that is very unsatisfying for her.

65. Carol seems to have an abundance of ____ in her life.
    A. financial resources
    B. friends
    C. stress
    D. spare time

66. To alleviate her stress, Carol should consider:
    A. quitting her job and staying home with her children
    B. making up with her husband and not going ahead with their divorce
    C. making time to sit quietly each day and connecting with her spiritual self
    D. taking off for a few hours each day and not telling anyone where she is

67. When in the middle of a stressful situation, Carol should:
   A. leave the salon and not return until the next day
   B. take a couple of deep breaths to get herself centered
   C. blame the other person for what is happening
   D. decide to change careers and leave without notice

68. How is Carol currently handling her stress?
   A. She is becoming calm and not allowing the situation to bother her
   B. She is throwing things out of rage and frustration
   C. She is becoming impatient and snapping at others
   D. She is becoming anxious and too frightened to act

69. In order to handle her stress, Carol may need to create more ___ in her life.
   A. balance
   B. instability
   C. job opportunities
   D. dating options

70. In order to reduce her stress, Carol should try to:
   A. charge more for every service she performs
   B. get more sleep
   C. find a new caregiver for her children
   D. take an advanced cutting class

71. Which of the following could Carol do on a daily basis to relax?
   A. Go to the theater
   B. Go dancing with her best girlfriend
   C. Take a walk
   D. Buy a new outfit

Johnnie recently began working as an educator for a wet goods company. He travels every day from salon to salon, introducing products to stylists and teaching them how to use them. Johnnie's job is sometimes frustrating and hectic because he is always at the mercy of the salon manager as to whether or not he will be allowed to do his work. While waiting for styling staff to become available, Johnnie often finds himself drinking coffee and munching on doughnuts, candy, or pretzels, and because he often finds himself rushing from one salon to another, he finds it easier to drive through fast-food restaurants than to plan and pack his lunch each day. Also, because he is so busy, he decided to drop out of the baseball league that he had played in with his pals for the past five years. At his last doctor's visit, Johnnie learned that he had gained more than 20 pounds, and he complained that he feels tired and sluggish all of the time. His doctor suggested that Johnnie reevaluate his current lifestyle and lose the weight that he has gained.

72. If Johnnie wants to improve how he is feeling, what should he do?
    A. Eat a diet of only vegetables
    B. Cut all of the carbohydrates out of his diet
    C. Eat a nutritionally balanced diet
    D. Add more fats to his diet

73. In order to lose the extra weight that he's gained, Johnnie needs to consider:
    A. skipping lunch each day
    B. adding some moderate exercise to his day
    C. skipping dinner each evening
    D. working out all day at the gym

74. In order to maintain a healthy weight, Johnnie will need to monitor:
    A. snacking on junk food
    B. salt grams
    C. water retention
    D. protein levels

75. When Johnnie is waiting for his potential clients to become available, which of the following could he be doing to relieve his frustrations and stress?
    A. Meditating
    B. Eating low-fat popcorn
    C. Making phone calls
    D. Catching up on e-mail

76. What percentage of his daily caloric intake should Johnnie be receiving from fat calories?
    A. 10%
    B. 20%
    C. 30%
    D. 40%

77. Which of the following would be a healthy choice for Johnnie to choose for lunch?
    A. A pizza topped with extra cheese and a sundae for dessert
    B. A low-fat sandwich on a multigrain roll with fresh fruit
    C. A couple of tacos, large fries, and a soft drink
    D. A large order of onion rings

YOUR PHYSICAL PRESENTATION

Marilyn is both a hair stylist and nail tech who works about eight hours a day servicing clients. When she is standing, she very often leans on one hip or the other, shifting her weight from one side to the other. When she is seated, she usually leans forward with her legs either crossed or tucked underneath her body. At the end of the day, she is often in pain: her legs and back are cramping and her arms, shoulders, and neck feel tired and strained. By the time she arrives at home, she hardly has enough energy to do some routine chores before plopping in front of the television set for the evening.

78. What does Marilyn's physical presentation indicate?
    A. Excellent personal style
    B. Poor posture
    C. Decreased ability to retain clients
    D. Incredible physical strength

79. To achieve and maintain a good standing posture, in what position should Marilyn's head and neck be?
    A. Level with her elbow
    B. Tilted forward at a 45-degree angle
    C. Level with the floor
    D. Tilted backward at a 45-degree angle

80. To relieve the tension in her shoulders, Marilyn should:
    A. scrunch them together
    B. level and relax them
    C. lift one higher than the other
    D. bring them in close to the body

81. When standing, in what position should Marilyn's spine be?
    A. Curved laterally
    B. Swayed to the left
    C. Swayed to the right
    D. Perfectly straight

82. A sitting posture that would alleviate Marilyn's back and neck pain would include:
    A. curving her back forward
    B. stretching her back from left to right
    C. keeping her back straight
    D. crossing her feet at the ankles

83. If it is necessary for Marilyn to bend forward, which part of her body should be bent?
    A. Neck
    B. Shoulders
    C. Back
    D. Hips

84. How can Marilyn make her work environment more ergonomically correct for herself?
    A. She can bend forward to reach her clients better
    B. She can adjust the client's chair
    C. She can ask the client to lean forward
    D. She can stand during all of the services

85. To relieve muscle fatigue from standing for long periods, Marilyn could try:
    A. standing on a cushioned mat
    B. wearing slippers
    C. taking aspirin at the beginning of each shift
    D. wearing stacked, high-heeled shoes

Chapter 4

COMMUNICATING FOR SUCCESS

COMMUNICATION BASICS

Victoria is out shopping when she sees a salon and decides to go in for some advice. Abe, the stylist who happens to be sitting behind the reception desk, asks if he can help her. "Yes," says Victoria. "I need some help with my hair." Abe smiles and says, "Sure, what kind of help do you need?" Victoria thinks for a moment and then points to her wilted style and replies, "Well, I don't know, I'm not really happy with it right now." Abe asks her if she is unhappy with the length or the style. She shakes her head no and then replies, "I guess I need something that will help me get and keep body in my hair." "You want something that will help you get and keep body in your hair?" asks Abe. Victoria nods her head and says, "Yes, an hour after drying and curling my hair, it's flat again." Abe grabs a couple of hair magazines from the counter and asks Victoria to find a photo that is closest to the finished look she desires. Once he sees her selection, he says, "I see, you want a bit of height at your forehead but not too much width at the temple area?" Victoria nods her head in agreement and Abe hands her a bottle of sculpting gel, which he explains, is useful when styling her wet hair and a super-hold hairspray to use once the hair is dry to get the lift in the front that she desires. Victoria thanks him for listening to her and taking the time to recommend products for her specific needs. Victoria pays for the products and takes one of Abe's business cards before leaving the salon.

86. When Victoria first walked into the salon, what had she neglected to do?
    A. Decide on a new hair style
    B. Check on the name of the salon
    C. Collect her thoughts
    D. Make an appointment

87. When Victoria told Abe that she needed help with her hair, how did Abe help her articulate her thoughts more clearly?
    A. By booking her for a perm
    B. By suggesting a new haircolor
    C. By recommending another style
    D. By asking her questions

88. How did Victoria clarify her desires to Abe?
    A. By referring to another client in the salon
    B. By showing him a photo in a magazine
    C. By pushing her hair into place and recreating her look
    D. By describing it in minute detail

89. When Abe describes the attributes of the style she has selected back to Victoria, he is using a technique called:
    A. passive listening
    B. articulating
    C. reflective listening
    D. communicating

90. Based on the exchange between Abe and Victoria, what is the outcome likely to be?
    A. Victoria will probably never return to the salon
    B. Victoria may return to the salon, but will not request Abe's services
    C. Victoria will probably try a brand new salon and stylist for her next service
    D. Victoria may return to the salon and request Abe's services

91. By going the extra mile to fully understand Victoria's needs, Abe was attempting to build a strong _____ .
    A. relationship
    B. client base
    C. pay base
    D. commission

THE CLIENT CONSULTATION

Dennis is in the planning stages of opening a new, full-service salon that will offer hair, nail, and skin care service. As he works with his contractor to make the space useable for his needs, Dennis plans a consultation area that is separate and private from the styling and service areas of the salon. Once Dennis leaves the meeting with the contractor, he begins to make a list of the things he will need to provide for the consultation space so he can prepare for the salon's opening.

92. Dennis plans to equip the consultation area with the following furniture:
    A. a reception desk
    B. styling stations
    C. comfortable chairs and table
    D. nail stations

93. Which of the following materials is NOT necessary for Dennis to provide during a client consultation?
    A. A telephone
    B. Swatch charts
    C. A portfolio of styles
    D. Hairstyling magazines

94. What type of atmosphere should Dennis provide for the room to be most conducive while speaking to clients about their services?
    A. A room that is busy with the bustle of the salon
    B. A space that is dimly lit so that it is relaxing to the client
    C. A quiet, well-lit room so clients can adequately participate in the conversation
    D. A space that is central to color formulations and mixing

Dennis has opted to use the client card (Figure 4–7) for all of his salon's client consultations. Use the card as a basis for answering the following questions.

Client Consultation Card

Dear Client,

Our sincerest hope is to serve you with the best hair care services you've ever received! We not only want you to be happy with today's visit but we also want to build a long-lasting relationship with you—we want to be your hair care salon. In order for us to do so, we would like to learn more about you, your hair care needs, and your preferences. Please take a moment now to answer the questions below as completely and as accurately as possible.

Thank you, and we look forward to building a "beautiful" relationship!

Name: _____

Address: _____

Address: _____

Phone Number: _____ (day) _____ (evening) _____

Sex: _____   Male _____   Female _____   Age: _____

How did you hear about our salon?

If you were referred, who referred you?

Please answer the following questions in the space provided. Thanks!

1. Approximately when was your last salon visit?
2. In the past year, have you had any of the following services either in or out of a salon? (Please indicate the date on which you had it.)

   ____Haircut   ____Full Head Lightening
   ____Haircolor   ____Waxing (what type?)
   ____Permanent Wave or   ____Manicure
      Texturizing Treatment   ____Artificial Nail Services (please describe)
   ____Chemical Relaxing or   ____Pedicure
      Straightening Treatment   ____Facial/Skin Treatment
   ____Highlighting or Lowlighting   ____Other (please list any other services you've
                                               enjoyed at a salon that may not be listed
                                               here).

3. Are you currently taking any medications? (Please list)
4. What is your natural hair color shade?
5. How would you describe your hair's texture?
6. How would you describe your hair's condition?
7. How would you describe the condition of your scalp?
8. What type of skin do you have? Dry _____   Oily _____   Normal _____
   Combination _____
9. What type of skin care regimen do you follow? (Please explain) _____
   _____
10. How would you characterize your nails? Normal _____   Brittle _____   Flexible _____
11. Do you have any of the following nail services? (check all that apply) Silk wraps _____
    Porcelain _____   Acrylic wraps _____   Glue manicure _____
    Natural manicure _____   Paraffin hand treatments _____
12. Do you have any of the following foot services? (Check all that apply) Basic pedicure
    _____   Spa pedicure _____   Paraffin foot treatment _____
13. Do you ever experience dry, itchy skin?   Scalp?   If so, how often?
14. Do you notice that your ability to manage your hair, skin, or nail regimens change with
    the change in climate? How so?

(continued)

15. How often do you shampoo your hair?
16. How often do you condition your hair?
17. Once cleansed and conditioned, how do you style your hair?
18. Please list all of the products that you use on your hair, skin, and nails regularly.
19. On average, how much time do you spend each day styling your hair?
20. Are you now or have you ever been allergic to any of the products, treatments, or chemicals you've received during any salon service—hair, nails, or skin? (Please explain)
21. What is your biggest complaint concerning your hair?
22. What is your biggest complaint concerning your skin?
23. What is your biggest complaint concerning your nails?
24. What do you like about your hair?
25. What do you like about your complexion?
26. What do you like about your nails?
27. Please describe the best hairstyle you ever had and explain why you felt it was the best.
28. What is the one thing that you want your stylist to know about you/your beauty regimens?

NOTE: If this card was used in a beauty school setting, it would include a release form at the bottom such as the one below.

Statement of Release: I hereby understand that cosmetology students render these services for the sole purpose of practice and learning, and that by signing this form, I recognize and agree not to hold the school, its employees, or the student liable for my satisfaction or the service outcome.

Client Signature _____ Date _____

Service Notes

Today's Date:
Today's Services:
Notes:

Today's Date:
Today's Services:
Notes:

Today's Date:
Today's Services:
Notes:

Today's Date:
Today's Services:
Notes:

Today's Date:
Today's Services:
Notes:

Figure 4–7. Client Consultation Card

95. Having clients fill in all of the questions pertaining to their address and other personal information allows Dennis' salon to:
    A. sell a list of client information to other businesses
    B. correctly identify each client
    C. determine the number of dollars in sales they make each year
    D. keep clients even after a stylist leaves the salon

96. Knowing when the client last visited a salon will help the stylists in Dennis' salon to:
    A. determine how much return business can be expected from this client
    B. assess the client's commitment to her style's upkeep
    C. determine how much to charge for the service
    D. assess how much retail product to sell the client

97. Asking clients which services they have had in the previous year allows the salon to:
    A. assess the number of times they cut their own hair
    B. determine if they can afford more services this year than last
    C. identify the chemical treatments with which the clients have been happy
    D. determine the client's history and the hair's condition

98. Why is it useful for Dennis to ask clients about the medications they take?
    A. So he can notify the closest pharmacy
    B. So he can prescribe additional medications
    C. So he can assess the effect of the medication on their beauty regime
    D. So he can notify their physicians of the services he will perform

99. Dennis requires clients to answer questions about their skin and nail care because:
    A. he is opening a full-service salon
    B. he is opening a nail salon
    C. he is opening a haircolor salon
    D. he is opening a luxury spa

100. Why is it important for Dennis to know how often clients wash and condition their hair?
    A. So he can recommend a pricey shampoo for them to purchase
    B. So he can determine their hair care routine and suggest services that will work for them
    C. So he can recommend a pricey conditioner for them to purchase
    D. So he can give them a second shampoo before beginning his service to really cleanse their hair

101. Asking clients about their allergies allows Dennis to:
    A. protect staffers from allergic reactions
    B. prescribe appropriate treatments
    C. protect clients from products or services that may harm them
    D. find holistic treatments to cure clients' allergies

102. Which of the following is exactly the type of information Dennis' stylists should include in the Service Notes section of the consultation card?
    A. Any notes pertaining to the client's personality during the service
    B. Any notes pertaining to the client's sense of humor during the service
    C. Any notes pertaining to the client's clothing during the service
    D. Any notes pertaining to the client's hair or its reaction during the service

SPECIAL ISSUES IN COMMUNICATION

Angie has been referred to Marshall by a friend who is one of Marshall's long-time clients. Angie loves the way he cuts and styles her friend's hair, and she is eager to meet Marshall and have him cut and style her hair. Angie shows up on time for her appointment. When she arrives at the salon, she finds a lot of people and confusion in the reception area. Since she has never visited this salon before, she is unsure of what to do. Angie approaches the reception desk and tells the person seated behind the desk her name and the name of the stylist with whom she has an appointment. The receptionist nods her head and turns her back to Angie to answer the telephone. Angie sits down and waits for Marshall. A few minutes go by and a young woman comes down to the waiting area, picks up a slip of paper, calls Angie's name, then turns and goes toward the shampoo area. Angie stands up but the young woman is already gone. Angie again approaches the reception desk and asks what she should do. The receptionist tells her to follow the woman, who is Marshall's assistant, to the shampoo station so she can be shampooed and prepared for Marshall. Angie rushes through the styling floor and finally sits down in a shampoo chair. After her hair is shampooed, Angie is led to a styling station and told to sit down. Another couple of minutes pass when finally, a young man walks over to Angie. He begins to towel dry her hair and says, "What can I do for you today?" Angie, confused, asks if he is Marshall. He smiles and sarcastically replies, "Well, I was when I got in here this morning!"

103. Based on this scenario, Angie's first impression of the salon is likely to be that it is:
    A. extremely professional and concerned with making new clients feel welcomed
    B. disorganized and too confused to make a new client feel comfortable
    C. extremely professional but too confused to make a new client feel comfortable
    D. disorganized but concerned with making new clients feel welcomed

104. How should Marshall's assistant have greeted Angie?
    A. Exactly as she did
    B. With a smile and a handshake
    C. With a solemn look on her face
    D. With a joke about the weather

105. When Angie arrived at the salon and checked in, what should the receptionist have offered to do?
    A. Park her car for her
    B. Change the music station on the radio
    C. Give her a tour of the salon
    D. Introduce her to the owners

106. Although the salon was obviously busy, what could Marshall's assistant have done to help direct Angie?
    A. Get her shampooed and into the styling chair as soon as possible
    B. Wait for Angie to get up and accompany her to the shampoo area
    C. Call to her from the shampoo area
    D. Skip the shampoo and taken her directly to the styling chair

107. What should have been the first thing that Marshall said to Angie when he approached her?
    A. "Hi, my name is Marshall. Welcome to the salon."
    B. "How much would you like me to trim off your hair?"
    C. "I'm running a bit behind: do you need to have your hair shampooed?"
    D. "Did anyone explain how we charge for our services?"

HANDLING TARDY CLIENTS

It is a particularly busy day at the Newmark Salon where Susan works as a nail tech. Today, a loyal salon client, Kim, has several appointments scheduled beginning with a manicure appointment at 1 P.M. After the manicure, she is scheduled for an eyebrow waxing at 1:45 P.M. and a haircut at 2 P.M. Since Susan is booked with appointments all day long, and since at 1:20 P.M. Kim still hadn't arrived, Susan decides to start her next client, Mrs. Trevino. At 1:30 P.M. Kim came into the salon. When she was told by the receptionist, Patti, that she was late for her nail appointment, Kim argued that she had made the appointment for 1:30 P.M. and was on time.

108. Patti should handle the scheduling mixup by:
    A. proving that she was right and Kim was wrong
    B. interrupting Mrs. Trevino's service and having Susan begin Kim's service
    C. asking Kim to visit another salon in the future
    D. apologizing for the mixup and offering to reschedule the appointment

109. If Kim insists that she needs her nail appointment today, what can Patti do to accommodate her request?
    A. Tell Kim that since she was late, there is nothing that can be done
    B. Check with Susan and reschedule Kim for an appointment at the end of the day
    C. Make a nail appointment for her at another salon
    D. Cancel all of her appointments for today

110. In regard to Kim's remaining appointments, the salon should:
    A. be able to accommodate her eyebrow waxing and haircut appointments as scheduled
    B. reschedule her haircut appointment
    C. demand that she reschedule all of the day's appointments
    D. reschedule her eyebrow waxing appointment

111. If Kim is upset about not being able to have her nail service immediately, Patti should refer her to:
    A. another salon
    B. the salon's employee policy
    C. another receptionist
    D. the salon's late policy

112. What could the salon easily do to confirm appointments for clients the evening before their appointments?
    A. Mail reminder notices
    B. Call clients and confirm appointments
    C. Fax special stylist announcements
    D. E-mail clients additional services descriptions

Ruth has just cut Mrs. Mendez's hair for the first time. She felt that she really understood Mrs. Mendez's directions and requests, but now that she has completed the cut and blow-dry service, her client is very unhappy and has begun to cry. Ruth is understandably nervous and upset herself, but she knows that she must address Mrs. Mendez's concerns quickly so as not to upset other salon clients.

113. Where is the best place for Ruth to have the conversation with Mrs. Mendez about what is wrong?
    A. At her styling station
    B. In the reception area
    C. At the shampoo bowl
    D. In the consultation area

114. Which of the following most closely resembles a question that Ruth should be asking Mrs. Mendez?
    A. "Would you like to have a free conditioning treatment?"
    B. "Would you like a cup of coffee?"
    C. "What specifically don't you like about the style?"
    D. "Would you like to book now for a perm next month?"

115. If Ruth is able to determine from Mrs. Mendez that she would prefer more layers cut into the style, what should Ruth do?
    A. Cancel her next appointment and recut Mrs. Mendez's hair
    B. Tell Mrs. Mendez to remember what she wants the next time she gets her hair cut
    C. Note Mrs. Mendez's complaints on her client consultation card and file it promptly
    D. Schedule Mrs. Mendez for the next available appointment and recut her hair

116. In the areas around the head where it is already too short and more layers can't be cut into the style, Ruth must:
    A. pretend to cut those areas to match the others
    B. act as if they are not a part of the finished style
    C. honestly tell the client that they cannot be reshaped
    D. cut them shorter and hope that they blend in with the new cut

117. If Ruth is not able to determine the source of Mrs. Mendez's dissatisfaction and they are not able to come to an amiable resolution, Ruth should:
    A. call on her manager or a senior stylist for help and advice
    B. make an appointment for her at another salon
    C. give her a gift certificate for a year of free services
    D. ask her to leave and never return to the salon

118. How can Ruth use this experience to grow as a professional stylist?
    A. She can use the feedback to improve her service for the next client
    B. She can use the experience as confirmation that she is in the wrong industry
    C. She can use the feedback to blame the miscommunication entirely on the client
    D. She can chalk up the experience to having had a bad day

IN-SALON COMMUNICATION

Myrna has just joined the Master Hair Salon where Bonnie and Stacy have been working for more than a year. Recently, while Stacy was on vacation, Bonnie serviced one of her long-time clients and gave her some advice about her haircolor that differed from the advice Stacy had given her, and she was more satisfied now with her color service than she previously had been. Now, the client has become a regular client fan of Bonnie's, and Stacy has accused Bonnie of deliberately trying to steal her clients away. The argument has turned ugly in that each is gossiping about the other to their salon coworkers and clients, and the stress of this on-going feud has caused a lot of tension in the salon. As the new person, Myrna has been approached by each stylist, and now must decide how to proceed in this environment.

119. Myrna's best course of action is to:
    A. keep her clients away from Bonnie
    B. treat both stylists respectfully and fairly
    C. keep her clients away from Stacy
    D. treat both stylists with contempt and distrust

120. When asked whose side Myrna believes, she should:
    A. decide that she believes Stacy and ignore Bonnie
    B. remain partial to Bonnie
    C. decide that she believes Bonnie and ignore Stacy
    D. remain neutral

121. If pushed into the conflict, what should Myna say to Bonnie and Stacy?
    A. "I don't like or believe either one of you."
    B. "I am really ashamed at how childish you two are acting"
    C. "I think you are both terrible stylists and I would have advised the client totally differently"
    D. "I like you both and don't want to be involved in your argument"

122. If Myrna continues to feel pressured about taking a side, her best course of action is to ask ___ for help in resolving the matter.
    A. her parents
    B. her salon manager
    C. her best friend
    D. her boyfriend

123. If Myna is feeling victimized about the pressure to get involved in the salon conflict, she may feel tempted to discuss it with other salon staff which would be:
    A. an excellent way to get to know others in the salon
    B. detrimental to maintaining a professional relationship at work
    C. a good way to hear what the other stylists think of the conflict
    D. an easy way to get around talking to Bonnie and Stacy

It is October and Bruce realizes that he will be having a meeting with his manager, Jackie, to review his employee evaluation. He hopes to hear that he is doing well at the salon, and he hopes to discuss some thoughts and ideas he has with Jackie as well. One thing on Bruce's mind is the construction that is occurring in front of the salon and how he feels that it is discouraging the salon's walk-in business. Another issue he hopes to discuss is the flex time policy the salon has adopted because he isn't sure how it should be affecting the late evening shift that he usually ends up working alone. And finally, he wants to talk to Jackie about the possibility of working toward a promotion to assistant manager of the salon.

124. In preparation for the evaluation meeting, Bruce should think about and list:
A. why he should get a larger raise than the other stylists
B. all of the problems in the salon
C. problems and possible solutions
D. the ways in which he is a better stylist than his coworkers

125. When discussing the issue of the construction outside of the salon and its effect on the salon's walk-in business, Bruce should:
A. show Jackie how much money the salon is losing because of it
B. calculate how many clients are leaving the salon because of the noise
C. stand at the door and count how many new clients walk by the salon in a day
D. suggest some ideas for how to work around the inconvenience of the construction

126. When discussing the flex time policy and the fact that he is often left at the salon alone in the evening, Bruce needs to:
A. complain that it isn't fair
B. list all of the names of stylists who have left early when they shouldn't have
C. make the case for his appointment to night manager
D. ask for an explanation of the policy and how it should affect the evening shift

127. When discussing any opportunities there may be for promotion, Bruce will need to be prepared to hear:
     A. that he can have the job
     B. the areas that he will need to improve in order to be considered for a promotion
     C. that someone else has already asked for the promotion
     D. the budget restrictions disallow for another assistant manager position

128. If Bruce is serious about working toward a promotion, he will want to ask Jackie:
     A. when they can meet again to discuss his progress
     B. if he can begin to work part time
     C. why she hasn't considered him for a promotion before now
     D. when he can expect to be made a salon partner

129. Once the evaluation is completed, Bruce should ____ Jackie
     A. thank
     B. flatter
     C. praise
     D. ignore

Part II—COSMETOLOGY SCIENCES

Chapter 5

INFECTION CONTROL: PRINCIPLES AND PRACTICE

BACTERIA

Mark and Cathy both work at the Sole Salon and Spa and their stations are right next to one another. Mark's daughter Maureen has been diagnosed with strep throat and has been home from school sick for several days. The following week, both Cathy and one of Mark's clients, Jane, are also diagnosed with strep throat after seeing Mark for a haircut.

1. Mark appears to be spreading bacteria called:
   A. cocci
   B. streptococci
   C. diplococci
   D. staphylococci

2. How might Cathy have been exposed to the bacteria that caused strep throat?
   A. By having a cup of coffee at work
   B. By breathing the same air as Mark
   C. By cleaning out her refrigerator at home
   D. By taking out the salon's trash

3. Bacteria that is disease-causing is called:
    A. pathogenic
    B. nonthreatening
    C. nonpathogenic
    D. threatening

4. Strep throat is:
    A. an organism
    B. a germ
    C. a secretion
    D. an infection

5. When Cathy looks inside of her mouth, she can see ____, which indicates that she has an infection.
    A. spirilla
    B. mitosis
    C. pus
    D. flagella

6. Mark should:
    A. assume that he is not spreading the disease and continue to work as usual
    B. stay home from work to protect the spread of disease
    C. assume that he is not spreading the disease but stay at home to be safe
    D. stay home from work to protect himself from becoming ill

7. A disease that can spread from Maureen to Mark to Cathy is said to be:
    A. advantageous
    B. communicable
    C. disadvantageous
    D. communicative

VIRUSES

Marlene and Sophia work together. Recently, Marlene has been feeling like she has the flu and she notices that her skin is somewhat yellow in color. Sophia has not been feeling well either. She has been tired and has had some stomach cramps to contend with. Both Marlene and Sophia work a lot of hours each week and eat most of their meals out. While they each try to keep their apartments neat, because of their busy schedules, they often go several weeks without really being able to clean and disinfect their respective living spaces.

8. What type of virus does Marlene likely have?
   A. HIV
   B. Hepatitis A
   C. AIDS
   D. Hepatitis C

9. What type of virus does Sophia likely have?
   A. HIV
   B. Hepatitis A
   C. AIDS
   D. Hepatitis C

10. How is Marlene's virus usually spread?
    A. By sharing an unsanitary restroom
    B. By borrowing money from another person
    C. From eating uncooked pork
    D. From bathing in a stream

11. How is Sophia's virus usually spread?
    A. By having sexual relations with an infected person
    B. By going to the movies with an infected person
    C. By loaning an infected person her hairbrush
    D. By shaking hands with an infected person

12. What organ is primarily affected by hepatitis?
    A. The heart
    B. The lungs
    C. The liver
    D. The spleen

13. Which of the diseases listed below can be treated with a vaccine?
    A. HIV
    B. Hepatitis A
    C. AIDS
    D. Hepatitis C

14. The disease-causing bacteria that are carried through Sophia's body are called:
    A. blood-loving pathogens
    B. bloodless pathogens
    C. bloodborne pathogens
    D. blood-using pathogens

15. In order to protect others from the diseases they carry, both Marlene and Sophia should:
    A. immediately stop working
    B. immediately disinfect any implements that come in contact with their body fluids
    C. immediately stop working together
    D. immediately wash any implements that come in contact with their body fluids

PARASITES

Three of the five nail clients Thomas has seen today all have nails with a strange, yellow-green spot just under the nail. His first client of the day, Marci, has the spot on her large toe, which he noticed while giving her a pedicure. Gina has a similar spot under a nail enhancement on her left hand and Bonita has a spot on her right hand. Marci is a waitress and likes to take good care of her feet. She has been a loyal pedicure client of Thomas' for the past five years. Gina, a swimming instructor, is a tried and true nail client, coming into the salon every two weeks for an acrylic fill. She has worn these nails for the last three years. Bonita, a schoolteacher, is a natural nail client who has a manicure and pedicure about once a month. When Thomas attempts to wipe away the discolored area, he is unable to.

16. What is the yellow-green spot that Thomas has detected likely to be?
    A. Dirt
    B. Infection
    C. Fungi
    D. Trapped water

17. Why can't Thomas remove the yellow-green spots he sees?
    A. Because they are a skin disease
    B. Because they are stained on the skin
    C. Because they can never be removed
    D. Because they must be cut off the nail

18. How could the fungus have been brought into the salon?
    A. Bonita may have caught it from one of her students
    B. Gina may have had moisture trapped under a nail
    C. Marci may have come into contact with spoiled food
    D. Thomas may have opened an expired bottle of acetone

19. How could the fungus have spread from one client to another?
    A. Improper disinfection of manicure implements
    B. By disinfecting the manicure table
    C. Improper sanitation of the nail enhancements
    D. By using the same nail polish wand on more than one client

20. What is the most common treatment for a nail fungus?
    A. Surgery to remove it
    B. Topical medication
    C. Constant washing of the infected area
    D. Spraying the infected area with disinfectant

IMMUNITY

Each year, Lucille and Frank, who are the coowners of the Serious Skin Care Center, take many precautions to ward off becoming ill during the cold and flu season. Frank makes it a habit to go to the doctor each year and get a flu shot because he knows that if he doesn't, he will undoubtedly get a cold or the flu at some point during the season. Lucille, on the other hand, makes a concentrated effort to take extra note of the vitamins she takes, to get a little extra sleep and relaxation, and to be sure to wash her hands frequently throughout the day, especially after servicing each client.

21. Both Lucille and Frank are attempting to enhance their ability to be ___ to/from disease.
    A. immune
    B. available
    C. susceptible
    D. contagious

22. Frank's flu shot is considered to be:
    A. a natural immunity
    B. a lost attempt at not getting sick
    C. a viable option for people who don't want to go to the doctor
    D. an acquired immunity

23. Lucille's ability to stave off the flu by taking excellent care of herself is an example of someone with:
    A. a natural immunity
    B. a lost attempt at not getting sick
    C. a viable option for people who don't want to go to the doctor
    D. an acquired immunity

24. Which of the following can be credited with promoting natural immunity?
    A. Eating raw meat
    B. Washing hands frequently
    C. Playing sports
    D. Taking long naps in the afternoon

PRINCIPLES OF PREVENTION

Jason is the new salon manager for the Good Looks Salon, and he is very concerned with the cleanliness of the salon and with preventing the spread of disease. In order to assess how the salon is doing in its efforts to control the spread of harmful disease and to make recommendations to his styling staff, Jason is about to review the salon's cleansing practices with the cleaning crew who has been hired to clean the salon each week. Ginger is the crew's supervisor, and she tells Jason that the salon is regularly disinfected and sanitized by use of chemical disinfectants such as quats, phenols and alcohol, and bleach, and with use of soap and detergents. Ginger also mentions that the cleaning crew follows all of the manufacturers' directions for use of all of these cleaning agents, and they follow OSHA guidelines.

25. In order to remove the pathogens and other substances that linger on the surfaces of the salon and on implements, the salon must be willing to:
    A. decontaminate
    B. bathe
    C. sterilize
    D. sanitize

26. When Ginger's crew disinfects the salon, they are using chemical agents to destroy bacteria and viruses on:
    A. facial skin
    B. cutting implements
    C. hair follicles
    D. nail clippings

27. Ginger's crew follow MSDS and OSHA guidelines, which tell them:
    A. how to enhance the fragrance of the product
    B. what time of day is best to use the product
    C. how to properly store and dispose of the product
    D. when to dilute the product for use on the skin

28. When Ginger considers the types of products for the crew to use, she must first decide if the product has the correct _____ for getting the job accomplished.
    A. audacity
    B. efficiency
    C. efficacy
    D. affection

29. The cleaning crew may use a quat because it is:
    A. effective in cleaning the scalp
    B. effective for cleaning under the fingernails
    C. effective for cleaning the windows
    D. effective for cleaning countertops

30. Jason can require the salon's stylists to use a ____ phenol solution for disinfecting metal implements.
    A. 5%
    B. 10%
    C. 15%
    D. 20%

31. Because it is not effective for use in the salon environment, which of the following forms of alcohol can't the cleaning crew use?
    A. Methyl
    B. Ethyl
    C. Anopropryl
    D. Isoproyl

32. The cleaning crews' ability to sanitize is limited mainly to the practice of:
    A. washing tools and implements with detergent
    B. cleansing countertops with quats
    C. disinfecting tables with phenols
    D. washing implements with alcohol

Keith is a busy cutter at Martin's Salon and Spa. Between each client, he quickly rinses his combs and brushes with warm water and drops them into a disinfecting solution. Keith allows them to become saturated, then reaches into the jar, pulls the implements out and wipes them dry with a towel, places them on his roll-about so he can access them easily before the next client is finished being shampooed, and has them delivered to his station by his assistant.

33. Before immersing his implements into the disinfecting solution, Keith should:
    A. immerse them in cool water
    B. wash them with soap and water
    C. blow-dry loose hair from them
    D. immerse them in boiling water

34. To protect himself, Keith should wear ____ when working
    with disinfecting solution.
    A. sneakers
    B. a cape
    C. a smock
    D. gloves

35. How should Keith mix the disinfecting solution?
    A. According to the salon owners' guidelines
    B. According to the salon managers' guidelines
    C. According to the manufacturers' guidelines
    D. According to the state boards' guidelines

36. How long should Keith's implements be immersed in the
    disinfecting solution?
    A. One hour
    B. Until the next client is ready
    C. As long as the directions recommend
    D. Four to six hours

37. By reaching into the disinfecting solution and pulling out
    the implements without using tongs or a glove, what is
    Keith causing to happen to the disinfecting solution?
    A. He is contaminating the solution
    B. He is doubling the effect of the solution
    C. He is sanitizing the solution
    D. He is diluting the strength of the solution

38. After the implements have been removed from the
    disinfecting solution, Keith should:
    A. store them at an empty station until he needs them
    B. place them in a clean, dry, disinfected container
    C. leave them rinsing in the shampoo bowl
    D. wrap them in a towel and put them in his drawer

Chapter 6

ANATOMY AND PHYSIOLOGY

CELLS

Malik has been feeling ill for quite some time when he finally decides to go to a doctor. The doctor performs a number of tests and diagnoses Malik with a disease that affects his cells' ability to remain healthy and reproduce.

39. Malik's cells contain _____ , a colorless, jelly-like substance in which food elements and water are present.
A. cytoplasm
B. protoplasm
C. nuclei
D. cell membranes

40. The nuclei of Malik's cells play a vital role in:
A. replication
B. repatriation
C. reproduction
D. reposition

41. If Malik's cells are unable to repair themselves, the problem most likely lies in the cells':
A. protoplasm
B. nuclei
C. cell membrane
D. cytoplasm

42. The two phases of metabolism that Malik's cells undergo are:
A. cannibalism and anabolism
B. catabolism and mitosis
C. catabolism and anabolism
D. anabolism and mitosis

TISSUES

In her training, Karen is studying the body's tissues and their uses. Since tissues are a collection of similar cells that all perform a particular function, Karen, in her work as an esthetician, knows that she will need to be aware of their affect on her clients, especially during services such as facials and massages.

43. The ____ tissue is responsible for supporting, protecting, and binding other tissues of the body together.
    A. nerve
    B. liquid
    C. connective
    D. muscular

44. The tissue that carries food, waste, and hormones through the body is called:
    A. nerve
    B. liquid
    C. connective
    D. muscular

45. As an esthetician, Karen will be very interested in the epithelial tissue since it includes the:
    A. feet
    B. senses
    C. skin
    D. scalp

46. When giving a facial massage, Karen will be coming into contact with the ____ system.
    A. nerve
    B. liquid
    C. connective
    D. muscular

47. When a facial client realizes that she feels relaxed and calm as a result of Karen's facial manipulations, it will be because the ____ tissues are carrying those messages from the brain to the rest of the body.
    A. nerve
    B. liquid
    C. connective
    D. muscular

ORGANS

Richard is losing his hair and realizes that for many reasons, especially esthetic reasons, he wants to do whatever he can to naturally slow the process. He speaks with his dermatologist who advises him to massage the top of his head, especially the areas where he sees the most hair loss, to eat a balanced diet, and to stop drinking soft drinks and replace them with plenty of water. His doctor also suggests that Richard begin taking long walks, take time to sit in peaceful places, and breath in clean air. Richard also realizes that because his skin is so dry, he should use a moisturizer to avoid skin breakage and cracking.

48. The organs most useful to Richard in realizing that he is losing his hair are the:
    A. kidneys
    B. eyes
    C. lungs
    D. stomach and intestines

49. When Richard is advised to massage his scalp, the doctor's intention is to increase Richard's blood circulation, which is a function of the:
    A. brain
    B. skin
    C. heart
    D. liver

50. Drinking plenty of clean water will allow Richard's body to eliminate waste products through the work of the:
    A. kidneys
    B. eyes
    C. lungs
    D. stomach and intestines

51. Supplying oxygen to the blood is the work of Richard's:
    A. kidneys
    B. eyes
    C. lungs
    D. stomach and intestines

52. Using a cream or lotion will moisturize Richard's skin, which is responsible for:
    A. removing toxins from his body
    B. controlling the body
    C. digesting food
    D. forming an external protective covering for the body

BODY SYSTEMS

Billy volunteers his time and his talent one day a week by going to a nearby nursing home and helping the residents by servicing their hair and beauty needs. Many of the residents at the home have very serious health problems. Although Billy knows he should never try to treat them, he is aware of the symptoms of their illnesses and able to notify the nurse on duty to watch out for the patient's well-being. On his schedule today are Mrs. Hammil, Mrs. Boxing, and Mrs. Reyper, all of whom want hair services.

53. While setting her hair, Billy notices that Mrs. Hammil's legs and ankles are swollen, which indicates that her _____ system is not working properly.
    A. circulatory
    B. digestive
    C. endocrine
    D. excretory

54. Mrs. Boxing has difficulty controlling the position of her head during her service; she is experiencing difficulty with her:
   A. digestive system
   B. muscular system
   C. endocrine system
   D. excretory system

55. During her perm, Mrs. Reyper sounds like she is having difficulty breathing. This is the work of the:
   A. endocrine system
   B. skeletal system
   C. excretory system
   D. respiratory system

THE SKELETAL SYSTEM AND THE MUSCULAR SYSTEM

Dennis is a businessman with a very stressful job. He has an appointment with Chris for a haircut, and decides to add on a scalp and head massage before his haircut. Dennis complains of head and neck aches to Chris and tells her that he isn't sleeping as comfortably as he would like.

56. In the first part of the massage, Chris will begin at the crown and work her way down to the ____, which is above the nape.
   A. mandible
   B. parietal bone
   C. maxilla
   D. occipital bone

57. The muscle that Chris will be massaging when she works on Dennis' crown and occipital area is the:
   A. frontalis
   B. occipitalis
   C. origin
   D. insertion

58. The bone that forms Dennis' forehead is called the:
     A. mandible
     B. frontal
     C. maxilla
     D. occipital bone

59. The muscle that allows Dennis to raise his eyebrows is the:
     A. frontalis
     B. occipitalis
     C. origin
     D. insertion

60. To relieve the tension at his temples, Chris will massage Dennis' ____ muscle.
     A. frontalis
     B. occipitalis
     C. temporalis
     D. insertion

61. The bones that are Dennis' temples are the:
     A. lacrimal bones
     B. parietal bones
     C. temporal bones
     D. occipital bones

62. To relieve his neck aches, Chris suggests that Dennis sleep with a soft pillow supporting the seven bones of his:
     A. nasal cavity
     B. thorax
     C. cervical vertebrae
     D. scapula

63. The muscle responsible for the movement of Dennis' neck and head is the:
     A. aponeurosis
     B. masseter
     C. platysma
     D. sternocleidomastoideus

Betty has been told time and time again by her clients that the best part of a manicure is the hand and arm massage. Today, she takes extra time with Pam, who is an administrative assistant and spends a lot of time on her computer, and Betty takes special care of her fingers and wrists.

64. When Betty massages Pam's fingers, the muscles that are responsible for separating the fingers are the:
A. flexors
B. triceps
C. abductors
D. adductors

65. While massaging Pam's fingers, Betty will be concentrating on massaging the bones of the:
A. ulna
B. carpus
C. phalanges
D. metacarpus

66. Because of her work, she is in danger of having pain in her:
A. ulna
B. carpus
C. phalanges
D. metacarpus

67. In order to massage the palm of Pam's hand, Betty would come into contact with the:
A. ulna
B. carpus
C. phalanges
D. metacarpus

68. The muscles in the palm of Pam's hand that enable her to move her thumb toward her fingers are called the:
A. flexors
B. opponent
C. abductors
D. adductors

69. Betty finishes Pam's treatment by massaging her upper arm, also called the:
A. ulna
B. humerus
C. carpus
D. phalanges

70. The muscle that allows Pam to rotate her palm outward is the:
    A. supinator
    B. biceps
    C. triceps
    D. extensors

Alma is a middle-aged facial client of the Skin Deep Salon and she asks her esthetician, Cindy, what she can do to help her tone and maintain the muscles of her face, especially, she sarcastically notes, around her mouth, eyes, and nose where she has begun to notice wrinkling. Alma wants to remain looking as young as she can without having cosmetic surgery. Cindy explains that there are several muscles in those areas that could benefit from gentle massage.

71. The muscle in Alma's forehead that is responsible for vertical wrinkles is the:
    A. masseter
    B. temporalis
    C. buccinator
    D. corrugator

72. The muscle between the cheek and upper and lower jaw that compresses the cheeks and gives Alma the appearance of high cheek bones is the:
    A. masseter
    B. temporalis
    C. buccinator
    D. corrugator

73. The muscle around Alma's eye socket that is toned so as to reduce the tiny wrinkles around her eyes is the:
    A. orbiculoaris oculi
    B. buccinator
    C. depressor labii inferioris
    D. corrugator

74. The muscle that causes wrinkles across the bridge of Alma's nose is the:
    A. orbiculoaris oculi
    B. procerus
    C. depressor labii inferioris
    D. platysma

75. When she made her sarcastic comment about looking young, Alma employed her ____ muscle to lower her lower lip and draw it to one side.
    A. orbiculoaris oculi
    B. procerus
    C. depressor labii inferioris
    D. platysma

76. The muscle that would allow Alma to draw her lips into a pout is the:
    A. orbiculoaris oculi
    B. procerus
    C. depressor labii inferioris
    D. levator anguli oris

THE NERVOUS SYSTEM

Sean is a very successful hairdresser who works hard to accommodate his clients' needs. He has recently read a number of articles about how important it is for truly successful people to take excellent care of their bodies as well as their minds. Sean spent some time thinking about this and evaluating his life, and he decided to commit to a regular exercise routine, going to the gym three times a week and eating a health-conscious diet. Sean's workouts involve lifting weights and working out on machines designed to build his strength. Sometimes, the workout routine leaves Sean out of breath and light-headed. For his protection, the gym requires Sean to frequently stop and check his heart rate, which is oftentimes elevated. Sean also sometimes experiences leg cramps in his sleep.

77. The system whose activities are responsible for Sean's thought processes about exercise is the:
    A. autonomic nervous system
    B. peripheral nervous system
    C. central nervous system
    D. astronomic nervous system

78. When Sean realizes that he feels tired as a result of his workout, the realization is the ____ system at work.
    A. autonomic
    B. peripheral
    C. central
    D. astronomic

79. When Sean's heart rate becomes elevated, it is the response of the ____ system to the workout.
    A. autonomic
    B. peripheral
    C. central
    D. astronomic

80. The type of nerves that carry the sensation of Sean's leg cramps to the brain are the:
    A. afferent
    B. different
    C. motor
    D. mixed

81. The nerves that carry the message from his brain to his muscles, thus allowing Sean to pick up and move weights during his workout, are called:
    A. afferent
    B. different
    C. motor
    D. mixed

NERVES OF THE HEAD, FACE, AND NECK

Stress can sometimes run high at the Stop Here Salon, which employs more than 20 stylists and is located in a busy strip mall. In order to relieve some of the tension from the hectic schedule, the salon manager, Jo, has decided to introduce a new technique called expression therapy during a staff meeting. When a stylist is feeling the stress of the day, he is encouraged to go to the break room, close the door, make funny faces in the mirror, take a deep breath, laugh at himself, then return to his styling station. All agree to give it a try. To start, Mark decides to pull his ears away from his face and bend them downward. Anne puts her index finger on the tip of her nose and lifts it up slightly. Missy follows by extending her lower lip and chin into a huge pout. Laughing, Matt raises his eyebrows, as if he has just been shocked or surprised by something terrible. Finally, when Patsy pushed her lower lip and chin out from her face, the whole group couldn't stop laughing. They all agreed that this technique would be a great stress reliever. Jo flashed a huge smile at the staff and ended the meeting.

82. When Mark pulls his ears away from his face and bends them downward, he is affecting the ____ nerves.
 A. nasal
 b. infratrochlear
 C. auriculotemporal
 D. infraorbital

83. When Anne puts her index finger on the tip of her nose and lifts it up slightly, she is affecting the ____ nerve.
 A. nasal
 B. infratrochlear
 C. auriculotemporal
 D. infraorbital

84. When Missy extends her lower lip and chin into a pout, she is affecting the ____ nerve.
 A. nasal
 B. infratrochlear
 C. mental
 D. infraorbital

85. When Matt raises his eyebrows as if he has just been shocked or surprised, he is affecting the ____ nerve.
 A. nasal
 B. supraorbital
 C. mental
 D. supratrochulear

86. When Patsy pushes her lower lip and chin out from her face, she is affecting the ____ nerve.
    A. zygomatic
    B. temporal
    C. buccal
    D. mandibular

87. When Jo flashes a huge smile at the staff, she is affecting the ____ nerve.
    A. zygomatic
    B. temporal
    C. buccal
    D. mandibular

THE CIRCULATORY SYSTEM

After running up and down the stairs from the salon's retail and reception area to the stock room where additional retail products are stored, John is completely out of breath and his heart is pumping hard.

88. The circulatory system consists of John's ____, arteries, veins, and capillaries.
    A. spinal cord
    B. heart
    C. reflexes
    D. mandible

89. Why is John's heart pumping so rapidly?
    A. To supply blood to parts of the body so he can have the energy to move about
    B. To remove too much blood from his heart, which prevents him from climbing stairs
    C. To move blood to his head so he won't be light-headed
    D. To pump additional blood into his nervous system

90. John's body is employing ____ circulation when it sends blood from the heart throughout the body and back to the heart again.
    A. pulmonary
    B. valve
    C. systemic
    D. capillary

91. John's heart is a:
    A. nerve
    B. artery
    C. tissue
    D. muscle

92. In order to purify it, John's heart will employ ____ circulation to send his blood to his lungs.
    A. pulmonary
    B. valve
    C. systemic
    D. capillary

93. The thick-walled muscular tubes that carry oxygenated blood away from John's heart to the capillaries are called:
    A. valves
    B. capillaries
    C. arteries
    D. veins

94. ____ are situated between the chambers of John's heart and they allow blood to flow in only one direction.
    A. Valves
    B. Capillaries
    C. Arteries
    D. Veins

95. John has ____, which are thin-walled blood vessels that are less elastic than arteries.
    A. valves
    B. capillaries
    C. arteries
    D. veins

96. John's ____ are minute, thin-walled blood vessels that connect the smaller arteries to veins.
    A. valves
    B. capillaries
    C. arteries
    D. veins

97. John's red blood cells:
    A. carry the body's cells to the heart
    B. carry cells to the blood
    C. carry cells to oxygen
    D. carry oxygen to the body's cells

98. John's white blood cells:
    A. destroy mold
    B. destroy harmful germs
    C. destroy useful bacteria
    D. destroy oxygen

99. The plasma in John's blood is responsible for:
    A. carrying food to cells
    B. carrying bacteria to cells
    C. carrying nerves to cells
    D. carrying muscle tissue to cells

100. Which of the following is NOT a function of John's lymph nodes?
    A. Provide waste to cells
    B. Carry nourishment from the blood to the cells
    C. Act as a defense against toxins
    D. Remove waste from cells

THE ENDOCRINE, DIGESTIVE, EXCRETORY, RESPIRATORY, AND INTEGUMENTARY SYSTEMS

Joan has recently begun to feel sudden and overwhelming rushes of heat, which she calls hot flashes. They are so severe at times that she has to stop servicing clients, excuse herself, and go into the restroom until they pass. After an episode, Joan is typically covered in perspiration and her clothes are wet. To help herself relax after such an episode, Joan practices deep breathing exercises that are designed to help calm her and return her heart rate to a normal and natural level.

101. The name of the system that affects the growth, development, and health of Joan's entire body is:
   A. circulatory
   B. endocrine
   C. respiratory
   D. digestive

102. Joan's endocrine glands secrete _____ into her bloodstream, which influence the well-being of her entire body.
   A. hormones
   B. bile
   C. urine
   D. carbon dioxide

103. The hormone most directly responsible for Joan's hot flashes is:
   A. insulin
   B. adrenaline
   C. estrogen
   D. testosterone

104. The _____, which is/are part of Joan's excretory system, is/are responsible for eliminating waste through perspiration.
   A. kidneys
   B. large intestine
   C. skin
   D. lungs

105. When she practices deep breathing exercises, Joan is employing her:
   A. kidneys
   B. large intestine
   C. skin
   D. lungs

106. The muscular wall that helps Joan control her breathing is the:
   A. lungs
   B. skin
   C. diaphragm
   D. diagram

107. When Joan breathes in and oxygen is absorbed into her bloodstream, the process is called:
    A. inhalation
    B. excretion
    C. exhalation
    D. urination

108. When Joan breathes out and carbon dioxide is expelled from the body, the process is called:
    A. inhalation
    B. excretion
    C. exhalation
    D. urination

109. Joan's skin, oil and sweat glands, sensory receptors, hair, and nails all belong to which of the following body systems?
    A. Circulatory
    B. Integumentary
    C. Respiratory
    D. Digestive

After a long day of servicing clients at the salon, Susan realizes that she hasn't eaten and feels very hungry. She decides to drive through a fast-food restaurant for a burger on her way home from the salon. She arrives at the order window at 9 P.M. and orders a hamburger, French fries, and a large iced tea. She pays for her food, then sits in her car and eats her dinner.

110. The system responsible for changing Susan's burger into nutrients and waste is the:
    A. circulatory
    B. endocrine
    C. respiratory
    D. digestive

111. Susan's ____ will be at work changing certain kinds of foods into a form that can be used by the body.
    A. insulin
    B. adrenaline
    C. enzymes
    D. estrogen

112. If Susan eats her burger at 9:15 P.M., what time will it be when her body completes the entire digestive process?
     A. 10:15 P.M.
     B. 1:15 A.M.
     C. 3:15 A.M.
     D. 6:15 A.M.

113. The iced tea that Susan drinks will be metabolized by her kidneys and will leave her body in the form of:
     A. bile
     B. perspiration
     C. urine
     D. carbon dioxide

114. Any food that is not decomposed will be eliminated by Susan's:
     A. kidneys
     B. large intestine
     C. skin
     D. lungs

Chapter 7

BASICS OF CHEMISTRY AND ELECTRICITY

CHEMISTRY

On his way into the salon for a full day of servicing clients, Jack realizes that he needs to fill his car with gas. He stops at a service station, fills his car's tank, purchases a small bottle of water and some chewing gum, pays for all of these, then heads for the salon. When he arrives, he finds that the sprinkler has just completed a cycle and the front of the salon is drenched with water. He steps over the puddles and walks into the salon. His first two clients are already there waiting for him: Mr. Ramirez, who will be having his hair cut and colored, and Ms. Crepa, who will be having a steam facial, a perm, and styling. With no time to waste, Jack gets to work.

115. The gasoline that Jack put into his car is considered to be:
    A. healthy
    B. organic
    C. unhealthy
    D. inorganic

116. Jack's gasoline is classified the way it is because it contains:
    A. power
    B. carbon
    C. oxygen
    D. energy

117. Jack's car, made of metal and steel, is considered:
    A. healthy
    B. organic
    C. unhealthy
    D. inorganic

118. The bottle of water that Jack bought is an example of:
    A. organics
    B. matter
    C. carbon
    D. inorganics

119. Jack's pack of chewing gum exists in ____ form.
    A. liquid
    B. element
    C. gas
    D. solid

120. The haircolor that Jack will apply to Mr. Ramirez is considered to be:
    A. an organic substance
    B. an example of matter
    C. an inorganic substance
    D. an example of carbon

121. The permanent wave solution that Jack will apply to Ms. Crepa is considered to be:
    A. an organic substance
    B. an example of matter
    C. an inorganic substance
    D. An example of carbon

122. Ms. Crepa's steam facial is an example of water in ____ form.
    A. liquid
    B. element
    C. gas
    D. solid

123. When Jack evaluates Mr. Ramirez's natural hair color level, he is determining its:
    A. chemical properties
    B. chemical composition
    C. physical properties
    D. physical composition

124. When Jack assesses the change in curl from before Ms. Crepa's perm to after it, he is assessing its:
   A. chemical properties
   B. chemical composition
   C. physical properties
   D. physical composition

125. When Mr. Ramirez's hair is cut, the change is considered to be:
   A. chemical
   B. physical
   C. gaseous
   D. elemental

126. When Mr. Ramirez's hair is colored, the change is considered to be:
   A. chemical
   B. physical
   C. gaseous
   D. elemental

PURE SUBSTANCES AND PHYSICAL MIXTURES

Nancy is booked for a full facial and makeup application, then a conditioning treatment and blow-dry at her favorite salon. She arrives at the salon and her facialist, Sierra, takes her right in and begins to perform the facial. First, she takes a powder from a sanitary bag and mixes it with water, applies it to Nancy's face, and lets it sit on the skin for three minutes. After removing this mixture, Sierra applies a facial scrub that is both smooth and rough because it contains small, hard particles scattered throughout. Next, she applies cold cream to Nancy's skin, which cools and soothes her face. Throughout the service, Sierra rinses her tools several times in water. When the facial is complete, Sierra shampoos Nancy's hair and applies the deep conditioning treatment. Once it was rinsed and her hair was dried and rolled on hot rollers, Sierra removes bottles and tubes of cosmetics and begins the makeup application with foundation. The foundation that she chose looked like it had separated in the bottle. Sierra shook it vigorously and then applied it to Nancy's face as a base.

127. The water that Sierra uses to rinse her tools is an example
of a:
    A. chemical compound
    B. physical compound
    C. solvent
    D. suspension

128. The foundation that Sierra used on Nancy's face during
the makeup application is an example of a:
    A. chemical compound
    B. physical compound
    C. solvent
    D. suspension

129. When Sierra blended the powder and the water for
application to Nancy's skin, she made a:
    A. problem
    B. mixture
    C. solution
    D. liquid

130. The powder that Sierra blended into the water is
considered to be a:
    A. solvent
    B. chemical compound
    C. solute
    D. suspension

131. The liquid into which Sierra blended the powder is
considered to be a:
    A. solvent
    B. chemical compound
    C. solute
    D. suspension

132. The fact that the water and powder mixed together
without separating implies that they are:
    A. united
    B. miscible
    C. opposed
    D. immiscible

133. Since the foundation that Sierra used had to be shaken every time it was used because the two compounds kept separating, it is an example of a/an ____ substance.
    A. united
    B. miscible
    C. opposed
    D. immiscible

134. The facial scrub that Sierra applied to Nancy's skin is an example of a ____ because it contains solid particles distributed throughout a liquid form.
    A. solvent
    B. chemical compound
    C. solute
    D. suspension

135. The hair conditioner that was applied to Nancy's hair is an example of a/an:
    A. water-in-oil emulsion
    B. color-in-water emulsion
    C. water-in-color emulsion
    D. oil-in-water emulsion

136. The cold cream that was applied to Nancy's skin is an example of a/an:
    A. water-in-oil emulsion
    B. color-in-water emulsion
    C. water-in-color emulsion
    D. oil-in-water emulsion

COMMON PRODUCT INGREDIENTS

Mike is creating an order list of products the salon needs to replenish when Allie, their distributor sales representative, comes into the salon next week. Every day, Mike adds to the list and he has asked all of his fellow stylists to add on items as they notice them becoming depleted. The list currently contains the following: rubbing alcohol, chemical hair relaxer, three jars of hand and skin cream for the manicure tables, hairspray, and water-resistant sunblock for retailing.

137. Mike's colleagues like using an alcohol that evaporates quickly for their needs in the salon. This type of alcohol is called:
     A. violent
     B. peaceful
     C. volatile
     D. passive

138. Which of the items on the list above is a form of ammonia?
     A. Hairspray
     B. Alcohol
     C. Sunblock
     D. Chemical hair relaxer

139. Which of the items on the list above contain glycerin?
     A. Hairspray
     B. Alcohol
     C. Hand cream
     D. Chemical hair relaxer

140. Which of the items on the list above contain silicones?
     A. Hairspray
     B. Alcohol
     C. Sunblock
     D. Chemical hair relaxer

141. Which of the items on the list above contain volatile organic compounds (VOCs)?
     A. Hairspray
     B. Alcohol
     C. Sunblock
     D. Chemical hair relaxer

It is another busy day in Marco's salon. He already has two of his clients in the reception area waiting their turns for services. The first, Barbra, has an appointment for a shampoo, condition, and updo, and Mandy, his second appointment of the day, is booked for a chemical hair straightening. As he reviews his scheduled appointments, he sees that he has a 1 P.M. appointment with Andrea for haircolor and a 2:30 P.M. appointment with Renee for a perm. Since he has so many chemical services to perform today, Marco takes a moment to remind himself of the issues surrounding pH and to picture the pH scale in his head.

142. When shampooing Barbra's hair, Marco will use water, which has a pH of:
  A. 3
  B. 5
  C. 7
  D. 9

143. The pH of the water Marco will use is considered to be:
  A. acidic
  B. alkaline
  C. potential
  D. neutral

144. The pH of Barbra's hair and skin is:
  A. 3
  B. 5
  C. 7
  D. 9

145. The pH of Barbra's hair and skin is considered to be:
  A. acidic
  B. alkaline
  C. potential
  D. neutral

146. Plain water is ____ than Barbra's hair and skin:
  A. 100 times less acidic
  B. 100 times more acidic
  C. 100 times less alkaline
  D. 100 times more alkaline

147. The chemical hair relaxer treatment that Mandy will receive will have a pH that indicates it is:
  A. acidic
  B. alkaline
  C. potential
  D. neutral

148. An alkaline pH is useful in straightening Mandy's hair because it will:
     A. harden and contract the hair
     B. soften and condition the hair
     C. harden and break the hair
     D. soften and swell the hair

149. When Marco performs his perm service later in the day for Renee, the perm will have a pH that indicates it is:
     A. acidic
     B. alkaline
     C. potential
     D. neutral

150. An acidic pH is useful in perm waving hair because it will _____ Renee's hair.
     A. harden and contract
     B. soften and condition
     C. harden and break
     D. soften and swell

151. After relaxing Mandy's hair, Marco will use a normalizing lotion that will neutralize the relaxer by creating a:
     A. relaxer-neutralizer reaction
     B. perm-neutralizer reaction
     C. acid-alkaline reaction
     D. oxidation-reduction reaction

152. When Marco's haircolor client, Andrea, has her service, he will witness a/an:
     A. relaxer-neutralizer reaction
     B. perm-neutralizer reaction
     C. acid-alkaline reaction
     D. oxidation-reduction reaction

153. If, when perming Renee's hair, an element is combined with oxygen, _____ will be produced.
     A. curl
     B. straightness
     C. heat
     D. odor

154. If heat is released during her perm, Renee's hair is experiencing an ____ reaction.
    A. endothermic
    B. combustible
    C. exothermic
    D. oxidizing

ELECTRICITY

Carlene has just parked her car in the salon's parking lot and realizes that because it has begun to rain, she will need to run to the salon's door to protect her beautiful new silk blouse from rain droplets. As she gets to the doorway, she realizes that she is the first person to arrive at the salon and will need to unlock the door. Once the door is opened, she steps into the salon's lobby and fumbles for the light switch in the dark. Finally, she puts the lights on, closes the door, and gets ready for the day. The first thing Carlene does is plug in her battery-operated curling iron so she can use it on her clients without worrying about it losing its power, and she plugs in her straight irons as well. Next, she makes sure that her cordless electric clipper is in its charger and finally, goes into the back room to make a pot of coffee.

155. Carlene's car employs a constant, even-flowing current, generated by a battery, which is called:
    A. in and out current
    B. constant current
    C. direct current
    D. alternating current

156. The form of energy Carlene was fumbling to activate when she entered the salon is called:
    A. reactions
    B. electricity
    C. electrotherapy
    D. light therapy

157. An ____ is what accounts for the lights coming on when Carlene flipped the switch.
     A. electric switch
     B. electronic handle
     C. electric current
     D. electronic current

158. Supporting the switch that Carlene turned on is a/an ____, which conducts electricity.
     A. insulator
     B. nonconductor
     C. conductor
     D. converter

159. Carlene's silk blouse is a:
     A. complete circuit
     B. nonconductor
     C. conductor
     D. converter

160. When Carlene plugs her travel curling iron into the wall outlet, she is using an apparatus known as a:
     A. rectifier
     B. converter
     C. complete circuit
     D. nonconductor

161. When Carlene plugs her straight irons into the wall outlet, she is using:
     A. in and out current
     B. constant current
     C. direct current
     D. alternating current

162. Carlene's cordless electric clippers are an example of a:
     A. rectifier
     B. converter
     C. complete circuit
     D. nonconductor

ELECTRICAL MEASUREMENTS

Martin intends to buy the Special Days hair salon, but before the deal is finalized, he has a walk-through with an electrical inspector, Andy, to be sure the salon is wired properly and able to handle the special electrical needs that a salon requires. They first inspect the outlets where the styling stations will be and where most of the hair drying and curling will take place. Next, they move to the facial rooms and discuss the special needs when giving facials. Finally, they move into the laundry room to inspect the area and outlets for a washing machine and dryer, and Andy explains the fuse box and circuit breaker.

163. Martin learns that normal wall sockets that power hair dryers and curling irons are _____ volts.
    A. 110
    B. 220
    C. 310
    D. 420

164. Outlets that can accommodate the correct amount of power for washing machines and dryers are _____ volts.
    A. 110
    B. 220
    C. 310
    D. 420

165. Andy explains that, due to its _____ rating, a hair dryer cord must be twice as thick as an appliance rated lower in order to avoid overheating and starting a fire.
    A. volt
    B. amp
    C. ohm
    D. watt

166. To create an atmosphere that is relaxing in the facial room, Martin will use a 40- _____ bulb.
    A. volt
    B. amp
    C. ohm
    D. watt

167. Martin's 2,000-watt blow-dryer will use ____ watts of energy per second.
    A. 2
    B. 20
    C. 200
    D. 2,000

168. If a fuse gets too hot and melts, Martin will know that:
    A. an appropriate amount of the current was prevented from passing through the circuit
    B. an excessive amount of current was allowed to pass through the circuit
    C. a deficit amount of current was prevented from passing through the circuit
    D. an excessive amount of current was prevented from passing through the circuit

169. If too many appliances are operating on the same circuit and they all suddenly stop working, Martin will know that the ____ has shut off to protect the salon from a dangerous situation.
    A. fuse
    B. amp
    C. circuit breaker
    D. watt

ELECTROTHERAPY

Karen is booked for a series of facial treatments with Gale, an experienced esthetician at the Red Tree Spa. Karen has some oil and blackheads trapped in the skin on her nose, and she has some dry patches on her cheeks and temple area. Karen would like to improve the muscle tone of her face and neck, increase the blood circulation, and relieve her congestion. Gale explains to Karen that she will be using various forms of electrotherapy in her treatments including galvanic current and faradic current, both of which are perfectly safe and useful in treating Karen's problems when administered carefully. Karen agrees and they begin the treatment.

170. Gale has prepared an electrode which is an ____ for use in treating Karen.
    A. applicator
    B. charger
    C. outlet
    D. plug

171. Gale determines that the positive electrode she will use, called the ____, is red.
    A. cathode
    B. charger
    C. anode
    D. plug

172. The first modality Gale will use is called ____ current, which is a constant and direct current.
    A. cathode
    B. galvanic
    C. plug
    D. faradic

173. If Gale wants to force acidic substances into Karen's skin, she must use:
    A. iontophoresis
    B. cataphoresis
    C. anaphoresis
    D. disincrustation

174. If Gale wants to force liquid into Karen's tissues, she must use:
    A. iontophoresis
    B. cataphoresis
    C. anaphoresis
    D. disincrustation

175. If Gale wants to introduce water-soluble products into Karen's skin, she must use:
    A. iontophoresis
    B. cataphoresis
    C. anaphoresis
    D. disincrustation

176. The process Gale will use to soften and emulsify the trapped oil deposits and blackheads on Karen's nose is called:
    A. iontophoresis
    B. cataphoresis
    C. anaphoresis
    D. disincrustation

177. In order to improve Karen's muscle tone, Gale will employ ＿＿current.
    A. tesla high-frequency
    B. galvanic
    C. sinusoidal
    D. faradic

178. In order to calm Karen's nerves, Gale will employ ＿＿ current.
    A. tesla high-frequency
    B. galvanic
    C. sinusoidal
    D. faradic

179. To relieve Karen of congestion, Gale will employ ＿＿ current.
    A. tesla high-frequency
    B. galvanic
    C. sinusoidal
    D. faradic

180. To increase glandular activity, Gale may use a ＿＿ on Karen.
    A. steamer
    B. heater
    C. vibrator
    D. conditioner

LIGHT THERAPY

After a couple of days off, Debbie has spent the day running around in the bright, hot sun completing errands, and she has just entered the salon she owns with her partner, Larry. Larry comments that she has gotten a bit of a tan and that it makes her look very healthy. He asks Debbie if she is ready for their meeting with Beth, their distributor sales consultant. They are going to discuss adding tanning services to their salon menu by putting a tanning bed in a small, unused room off the skin care area of their salon. Both Debbie and Larry have some concerns about the safety of tanning and are prepared to discuss them with Beth, who has just been to a training seminar and should have the answers they need to make the best decisions. Beth explains that tanning beds are safe as long as clients follow the manufacturers' instructions and guidelines, and that they provide both UV and infrared light. Beth also suggests that they consider using specialized light bulbs for treating some scalp and skin conditions.

181. The bright sunlight that Debbie experienced while running her errands is called:
   A. a wavelength
   B. invisible light
   C. therapeutic light
   D. visible light

182. Since Debbie has a slight tan, she has been exposed to:
   A. UV rays
   B. blue light
   C. infrared rays
   D. white light

183. To offer tanning services in the salon, Debbie and Larry must make sure that the UV rays are applied ____ inches from a light source.
   A. 10 to 16
   B. 20 to 26
   C. 30 to 36
   D. 40 to 46

184. Once the light source is correctly placed, it is safe, and Debbie and Larry's clients can have their first session under the light source. The first session should last ____ minutes.
    A. 1 to 2
    B. 2 to 3
    C. 3 to 4
    D. 4 to 5

185. Beth explains that infrared rays:
    A. produce the least amount of heat
    B. have the shortest wavelengths
    C. penetrate the deepest
    D. are the coolest

186. Beth explains that using ____ light is helpful for killing germs and should be used on bare skin.
    A. white
    B. yellow
    C. blue
    D. red

187. When Larry asks her about dry skin, Beth recommends using ____ light in combination with oils and creams.
    A. white
    B. yellow
    C. blue
    D. red

Part III—HAIRCARE

Chapter 8

PROPERTIES OF THE HAIR AND SCALP

STRUCTURE AND CHEMICAL COMPOSITION OF HAIR

Mrs. Brand is a very loyal client of the Hearts Salon. She colors and perms her naturally blond hair and makes a weekly visit to the salon for a wet set and comb out. On her most recent visit, Jean, her regular stylist, notices that Mrs. Brand's hair is very dry and rough looking.

1. When Mrs. Brand has her hair colored or permed, the chemical solution affects which layer of the hair shaft?
   A. Follicle
   B. Cuticle
   C. Cortex
   D. Medulla

2. If Mrs. Brand's hair looks and feels dry and rough, it is most likely a result of:
   A. contracting of the cuticle layer of the hair
   B. swelling of the hair's cortex
   C. contracting of the hair's cortex
   D. swelling of the cuticle layer of the hair

3. In order for her permanent haircolor and waving solution to actually change the hair's look, which layer of Mrs. Brand's hair must be affected?
    A. Follicle
    B. Cuticle
    C. Cortex
    D. Medulla

4. The appearance of Mrs. Brand's hair indicates that:
    A. the medulla has never been opened
    B. the cortex is completely closed
    C. the cuticle has been opened many times
    D. the follicle is completely absent

5. Based on the information you have on Mrs. Brand, it is very likely that her hair is missing a:
    A. follicle
    B. cuticle
    C. cortex
    D. medulla

6. Mrs. Brand's hair is made up of ____ protein.
    A. 19%
    B. 73%
    C. 91%
    D. 100%

7. When Mrs. Brand's hair is colored or permed, the bonds that are broken are called:
    A. protein bonds
    B. hydrogen bonds
    C. salt bonds
    D. disulfide bonds

8. When Mrs. Brand's hair is wet set, the bonds that are broken are called:
    A. protein bonds
    B. hydrogen bonds
    C. salt bonds
    D. disulfide bonds

9. When Mrs. Brand's hair is permed, the bonds that are broken are called:
   A. protein bonds
   B. hydrogen bonds
   C. salt bonds
   D. disulfide bonds

10. Mrs. Brand's natural blond hair is a result of the ____ in her hair's cortex.
    A. keratin
    B. eumelanin
    C. pheomelanin
    D. peptides

HAIR ANALYSIS

Marlene is a new client for John, so before he begins the cut and color service she has booked, he performs a hair analysis. While it is still dry, John looks at Marlene's hair and notes that she has what appears to be thick, curly, dark brown hair. When he touches her hair, it feels hard and glassy but slick and greasy, and he notices that she has a lot more strands of hair on her head than some of his other clients. On further investigation, John realizes that Marlene's hair grows in a circular pattern on the back of her head, at the crown. After her shampoo, John gently pulls Marlene's hair away from the scalp and sees that it readily springs back to its original place. John must now note all of his findings on his client record card before he begins to cut or color the client's hair.

11. In determining the texture of Marlene's hair, John notes that it is:
    A. fine
    B. medium
    C. soft
    D. coarse

12. Based on his diagnosis, Marlene's hair diameter and structure are characterized as:
    A. large and fine
    B. thin and coarse
    C. large and coarse
    D. thin and fine

13. John must be aware of Marlene's hair texture because it may affect the outcome of:
    A. whether he receives a large tip
    B. the haircolor service
    C. how many referrals Marlene will send to him
    D. the type of combs John will use while cutting

14. Based on what he felt when he touched her head, John noted that Marlene's hair density is:
    A. low
    B. medium
    C. moderate
    D. high

15. Marlene's hair density indicates that she has:
    A. only a few hairs per square inch on her head
    B. a medium number of hairs per square inch on her head
    C. a moderate number of hairs per square inch on her head
    D. a lot of hairs per square inch on her head

16. Based on Marlene's hair color, how many hairs is she likely to carry on her head?
    A. 140,000
    B. 110,000
    C. 108,000
    D. 80,000

17. Based on John's diagnosis of Marlene's hair, what is her hair's porosity likely to be?
    A. low
    B. normal
    C. average
    D. high

18. Chemical services performed on hair with Marlene's porosity require a/an:
    A. acid solution
    B. oxidative solution
    C. alkaline solution
    D. heated solution

19. Based on John's observations, Marlene's hair elasticity would be categorized as:
    A. low
    B. abnormal
    C. springy
    D. normal

20. The growth pattern that is evident on the back of Marlene's head is called a:
    A. stream
    B. whorl
    C. lake
    D. cowlick

21. John must remember Marlene's growth pattern, especially when:
    A. coloring her hair
    B. perming her hair
    C. spraying her hair
    D. cutting her hair

22. What type of hair and scalp condition does Marlene have?
    A. dry hair and scalp
    B. normal hair and scalp
    C. scaly hair and scalp
    D. oily hair and scalp

HAIR LOSS

Bonnie has just taken a new position at a salon that specializes in servicing clients with hair loss. On this particular day, she is booked with clients who have various forms of hair loss. Bonnie's first client of the day is Albert, a 70-year-old man whose hairline has receded about two inches but who otherwise has a thick head of healthy hair. Six months after having her baby, Anne, another of Bonnie's clients, is experiencing sudden hair loss. She is interested in having her hair cut short to make her daily routine easier and to minimize the appearance of the hair loss. Bonnie's final client of the day, a successful 40-year-old businessman named Martin, has just discovered a small round bald area at his nape and asks Bonnie to be sure to leave the hair above it long enough to cover that spot.

23. As she services Albert and learns about his hair loss, Bonnie realizes that his type of hair loss is categorized as:
   A. androgenic alopecia
   B. inherited alopecia
   C. alopecia areata
   D. postpartum alopecia

24. The cause of Albert's hair loss is likely to be his:
   A. styling regimen
   B. age
   C. shampoo
   D. water temperature

25. Anna's hair loss is categorized as:
   A. androgenic alopecia
   B. inherited alopecia
   C. alopecia areata
   D. postpartum alopecia

26. Anna's hair loss is usually:
   A. permanent with no more hair growth
   B. temporary with hair growth returning to normal within a year
   C. permanent with terminal new growth in three months
   D. temporary with only vellus new growth

27. Martin's type of hair loss is called:
   A. androgenic alopecia
   B. inherited alopecia
   C. alopecia areata
   D. postpartum alopecia

28. Martin's hair loss is caused by:
    A. brushing the hair too vigorously
    B. chemicals that were improperly applied
    C. an unpredictable autoimmune skin disease
    D. always wearing a baseball cap

DISORDERS OF THE HAIR AND SCALP

Judy has a full day of clients booked for various services. Her day begins with Mrs. Hines, who at 65 years of age has mostly gray hair with several areas of hair that are striped, both gray and dark. Joe, another of Judy's clients, wears his hair at a medium length, notes that his hair feels knotted, that he is experiencing lots of hair breakage, and is finding lots of small white flakes when he brushes or combs his hair. Joe's wife, Sandra, is also in the salon today. She is booked for an upper lip waxing because, she complains, she has dark, coarse hair on her face that almost looks like a man's mustache. When Jan arrives for services today, Judy asks one of the salon's assistants to shampoo her long hair and apply a deep penetrating conditioning treatment for 20 minutes to help her combat her spitting ends. On her day off, Judy will go to her son's third grade class and speak to the students about hair and scalp care, and she will warn them not to swap hats, especially if someone in the class may have head lice.

29. The technical term for Mrs. Hines' gray hair is:
    A. canities
    B. hirsuties
    C. monilethrix
    D. trichoptilosis

30. The technical term for Mrs. Hines' striped hair is:
    A. canities
    B. strained hair
    C. monilethrix
    D. ringed hair

31. The dark hair on Sandra's upper lip is a result of:
    A. canities
    B. hirsuties
    C. monilethrix
    D. trichoptilosis

32. The technical term for Jan's split ends is:
    A. canities
    B. hirsuties
    C. monilethrix
    D. trichoptilosis

33. The technical term for Joe's knotted and breaking hair is:
    A. monilethrix
    B. trichorrhexis nodosa
    C. trichoptilosis
    D. fragilitas crinium

34. The small white flakes Joe finds when brushing or combing his hair are called:
    A. tinea capitis
    B. scabies
    C. carbuncle
    D. pityriasis

35. The technical term for head lice is:
    A. tinea capitis
    B. scabies
    C. pediculosis capitis
    D. pityriasis

Chapter 9

PRINCIPLES OF HAIR DESIGN

PHILOSOPHY OF DESIGN AND ELEMENTS OF HAIR DESIGN

Andie has just returned from a terrific hair show where she attended several education classes and she is excited to use some of the techniques she learned there with her clients. One of the classes she attended was all about the elements of designing a great hairstyle that uniquely fit the needs and characteristics of the clients. Another class she took, a color class, described ways to use haircolor to enhance the clients face shape and hairstyle. The third class explored how wave patterns in the hair can be added or subtracted to further emphasize the shine and beauty of the hair.

36. Andie's excitement over what she learned at the hair show and her desire to try out some of the techniques is considered to be:
A. inspiration
B. depression
C. inertia
D. disinterest

37. When designing a style for hair that forces the eye to look up and down, Andie is creating a hairstyle with:
A. horizontal lines
B. vertical lines
C. diagonal lines
D. curved lines

38. Cathy, one of Andie's clients, is a single mom with three children who is looking for a very simple hairstyle that requires the least amount of care, so she must consider a:
A. single line hairstyle
B. repeating line hairstyle
C. contrasting line hairstyle
D. transitional line hairstyle

39. To create the illusion of a more slender face for her client Joan, Andie could use haircolor that is a:
    A. light color
    B. warm color
    C. dark color
    D. cool color

40. To create a hairstyle that reflects the most light for her client Meredith, Andie should consider a style with a ____ wave pattern.
    A. wavy
    B. curly
    C. very curly
    D. straight

PRINCIPLES OF HAIR DESIGN, AND CREATING HARMONY BETWEEN HAIRSTYLE AND FACIAL STRUCTURE

Since she was a teenager, Kim has worn the same hairstyle: long, dark, wavy hair that falls to just above the shoulders. Because she really wants to create a new look for herself, Kim makes an appointment with her stylist Courtney for a makeover. When she arrives, Kim talks with Courtney and explains what she sees as her problem areas. Kim complains that her face is too wide all the way around, that she feels she has a large forehead, that her eyes are set too close together, and that she has a wide, flat nose. Kim also feels that her hair is too wavy, and in order for her to keep it tamed, she has to wear her hair flat against her head, which she is bored with. Kim explains to Courtney that she wants to have a new style to accentuate her best features and minimize her flaws.

41. Based on Kim's description of her face, she has a/an ____ face shape.
    A. oval
    B. triangular
    C. round
    D. square

42. To help a round face shape appear longer and thinner, the best hairstyle is one that:
    A. is flat at the top of the head
    B. creates volume at the jaws and temples
    C. is close to the head all around with no volume at all
    D. creates volume at the top and is close at the sides

43. To minimize the appearance of Kim's forehead, Courtney should style her hair:
    A. away from the forehead
    B. across one side of the forehead
    C. back and off the face
    D. forward over the sides of the forehead

44. To combat her close-set eyes, Kim's hair should be:
    A. directed back and away from the temples
    B. directed forward and pointing to the eyes
    C. left long and hanging in front of the ear
    D. fringed over the ear and sculpted onto the face

45. What type of part is best for a face with a wide, flat nose?
    A. left side
    B. no part
    C. center part
    D. right side

46. To bring more definition to Kim's jawline, which type of line should be used?
    A. Rounded
    B. Wavy
    C. Straight
    D. Curved

47. When restyling Kim's hair, Courtney will need to make sure her wavy hair is _____ at the temple area and _____ at the top.
    A. close, high
    B. shaven, spiked
    C. high, close
    D. curled, straight

Chapter 10

SHAMPOOING, RINSING, AND CONDITIONING

UNDERSTANDING SHAMPOO AND CONDITIONERS

Alexia is a receptionist at the Bubbles Salon, and she is frequently asked to explain the various shampoos and conditioners and their uses to the clients who are serviced in the salon. She is surrounded by shelves full of products for retailing, and she answers questions and makes product recommendations all day long.

48. Barton is a 15-year-old client of the salon who frequently uses a lot of thick styling glue to get his hair into long spikes. He notices that his hair sometimes feels gooey even after shampooing. Alexia recommends a/an _____ shampoo for him.
    A. acid balanced
    B. conditioning
    C. medicated
    D. clarifying

49. Mrs. Kames is a long time haircolor client and needs a shampoo that will enable her to keep her color looking fresh between retouch visits. She should try a/an _____ shampoo.
    A. acid balanced
    B. color-enhancing
    C. medicated
    D. clarifying

50. Alexia usually suggests a client with _____ hair purchase a moisturizing shampoo.
    A. short
    B. permed
    C. roller set
    D. naturally curly

51. For Norman's oily scalp, Alexia suggests a _____ shampoo.
    A. balancing
    B. color-enhancing
    C. medicated
    D. clarifying

52. For Joyce, who washes, blow-dries, and hot curls her hair every day, Alexia recommends a _____ conditioner.
    A. rinse-through
    B. treatment
    C. leave-in
    D. repair

53. For Janice, who has a full head of bleached hair, Alexia recommends an in-salon conditioning service and a _____ conditioner for at-home use.
    A. rinse-through
    B. treatment
    C. leave-in
    D. color-enhancing

Chapter 11

HAIRCUTTING

BASIC PRINCIPLES OF HAIRCUTTING

Johnny is a master haircutter at a posh, upscale salon in town. He has spent many years perfecting his cutting skills and getting to know the human head form. Today, Johnny is booked solid. He has several clients to service and he is ready to get cutting!

54. Erin, Johnny's first customer, loves to wear an old haircutting favorite: the wedge. Johnny will use her occipital bone as his ____ for the entire cut.
    A. fringe
    B. reference point
    C. guideline
    D. cutting line

55. When cutting a client's hair for the first time, Johnny is careful to observe the ____ for unusual growth patterns such as cowlicks.
    A. top
    B. nape
    C. sides
    D. crown

56. When cutting long hair along the face to connect the bangs and the nape, Johnny often cuts a ____ line.
    A. straight
    B. vertical
    C. horizontal
    D. diagonal

57. When Johnny cuts Marianne's hair into a one-length bob, he uses ____ degrees of elevation.
    A. 0
    B. 45
    C. 90
    D. 180

58. Marianne's bob will be uniform if Johnny makes sure to continuously use his initial ____ guideline when cutting.
    A. stationary
    B. moving
    C. traveling
    D. layered

59. Darla has very long hair that she wants to be layered. To keep her hair long at the nape, Johnny cuts it by ____ the hair.
    A. blunting
    B. overdirecting
    C. thinning
    D. texturizing

CLIENT CONSULTATION AND TOOLS, BODY POSITIONS, AND SAFETY

Pat is looking over his appointment book today and sees that his first three clients will be in for haircuts. Lucy has very thick, coarse, straight hair. Frank has a good amount of hair that is easy to handle and moderately soft to the touch. Finally, Susan has thin, fine hair that usually lies limp no matter what style Pat cuts into it.

60. Lucy asks Pat what he thinks about her having her hair cut really short so it can just lay flat against her face. Pat explains that a cut like that will cause her hair to:
    A. fall out
    B. stand up away from the scalp
    C. become oily
    D. dry out

61. Which tool should Pat NOT use when cutting Lucy's hair?
    A. Sectioning clips
    B. Haircutting shears
    C. Razor
    D. Thinning shears

62. Frank likes to wear his hair short around the bottom and sides and fuller on top with a messy look. To achieve this, Pat will need to use _____ on the top.
    A. sectioning clips
    B. haircutting shears
    C. razor
    D. thinning shears

63. To get a clean line at the nape, Pat will employ a/an:
    A. razor
    B. clipper
    C. straight razor
    D. edger

64. To create the look of thicker hair, Pat needs to create _____ in Susan's style.
    A. layers
    B. weight
    C. partings
    D. thinning

65. The best cut for Susan's hair is the:
    A. graduated cut
    B. blunt cut
    C. layered cut
    D. long layered

66. The best cutting tool for Pat to use on Susan's hair is a:
    A. sectioning clip
    B. haircutting shears
    C. razor
    D. thinning shear

67. The type of comb that Pat will use for each of his haircuts will be the:
    A. side-toothed comb
    B. barber comb
    C. tail comb
    D. styling comb

CUTTING CURLY HAIR

Manny attends the ABC Beauty School and is enrolled in a cutting class for curly hair. Today, he and his classmates will cut and style three clients with varying amounts of curly hair. Manny's first client, Jenny, has very curly hair that falls down in ringlets. Jen wants her blunt cut trimmed so her hair will be about an inch shorter. Sandy, Manny's next client, has medium length wavy hair and she wants her new style to be shorter and chunky. Renee, his third client, wants to show off her curly hair, so she is looking for a mid-length style to showcase the curl.

68. To give Jen the trim she wants, Manny will need to:
    A. pull the hair taut to cut a straight line
    B. cut it straight across the bottom with no tension at all
    C. use an elevated guideline
    D. create layers with a 90-degree angle

69. To achieve the appearance of having cut Jen's hair one inch, Manny will actually need to cut off about:
    A. 1 inch
    B. ¼ inch
    C. 2 inches
    D. ½ inch

70. Cutting one inch of hair will make Jen's finished style appear ____ when it is dry.
    A. longer
    B. angled
    C. shorter
    D. diagonal

71. When Manny begins cutting Sandy's hair, he must be aware that her curly hair will need to be elevated ____ to achieve the desired look.
    A. more
    B. the same as straight hair
    C. less
    D. the same as color treated hair

72. To give Sandy's hair the chunky look she desires, he will need to texturize her hair using the ____ technique.
    A. thinning
    B. point cutting
    C. notching
    D. slicing

73. To give Renee the mid-length style she desires, Manny will need to cut the hair at a ____-degree angle all around the head.
    A. 0
    B. 45
    C. 90
    D. 180

74. To remove bulk and to add movement to Renee's cut, Manny will use a technique called:
    A. thinning
    B. point cutting
    C. notching
    D. slicing

Chapter 12

HAIRSTYLING

WET HAIRSTYLING BASICS, FINGER WAVING, PIN CURLS, ROLLER CURLS, AND COMB-OUT TECHNIQUES

Gayle has been styling hair for the movies for a number of years and she has recently been asked to work on a movie whose story takes place in the 1920s and 1930s. She will be responsible for styling the hair for the two lead characters, Esther and Johanna. The director explains to Gayle the look he is after for each of the characters. For Esther, he wants Gayle to create a real flapper look, with many wide but uniformly sized dark waves around the head. The hair should be close to the head when dry, perfectly curled into the wave formations, and set so that no matter how much dancing or movement the character experiences, the hair remains in place. The second character, Johanna, will need to wear her hair in a more flamboyant manner, so it should be light blond in color and the hair should sweep forward at the temples and onto the face. Johanna's hair requires lots of volume but the style should also be controlled and perfectly coifed so that it stays in place. Gayle begins working on her designs and the supplies she will need.

75. The list of supplies Gayle will need to have handy for styling the two characters include:
    A. scissors, comb, and hairspray
    B. blow-dryer, rollers, and comb
    C. scissors, blow-dryer, and clips
    D. clips, combs, and rollers

76. In terms of styling aids, Gayle will need to purchase:
    A. setting lotion, styling lotion, and hairspray
    B. setting lotion, mousse, and pomade
    C. styling lotion, hairspray, and leave-in conditioner
    D. styling mousse, spray wax, and hairspray

77. To achieve the close-to-the-head waves the director wants Esther to wear, Gayle will need to create:
    A. a wet set
    B. a layered cut
    C. a finger wave
    D. a pin curl

78. To ensure that Esther's hair lays appropriately for the style, Gayle should use:
    A. a left-hand part
    B. a part down the middle
    C. her natural part
    D. no part

79. The best type of comb for Gayle to use when creating Esther's style is a:
    A. tail comb
    B. styling comb
    C. wide-toothed comb
    D. barber comb

80. When Gayle completes styling Esther's hair, it should look like a continuous:
    A. B
    B. M
    C. S
    D. X

81. How should Gayle dry Esther's hair prior to combing it out?
    A. With a blow-dryer
    B. With a heat lamp
    C. With a Marcel iron
    D. With a hooded dryer

82. To create Johanna's style, Gayle will use:
    A. a blow-dryer, rollers, and pin curls
    B. a hooded dryer, round brush, and curling iron
    C. a blow-dryer, round brush, and flat iron
    D. a hooded dryer, rollers, and pin curls

83. To create the most volume she can on the top of Johanna's head, Gayle will place:
    A. rollers on base
    B. rollers off base
    C. rollers at half base
    D. rollers without a base

84. In order for Johanna's hair to sweep forward at her temples, Gayle will place pin curls into a/an _____ shaping.
    A. A
    B. B
    C. C
    D. D

85. In order to get a tight, long-lasting curl without too much mobility, Gayle will use:
    A. no stem pin curls
    B. full stem pin curls
    C. half stem pin curls
    D. part stem pin curls

86. To achieve a smooth, directed shape, Gayle will need to use a/an _____ base pin curl at the temple area of Johanna's style.
    A. rectangular
    B. triangular
    C. arc
    D. square

87. When combing out the finished style, Gayle will certainly need to _____ the hair on the top of Johanna's head to achieve the height she desires and to ensure the shape lasts as long as needed.
    A. back out
    B. back comb
    C. back cut
    D. back shape

BLOW-DRY STYLING AND TOOLS

Marcia has decided that after many years with the same styling tools and implements, she needs to purchase new, better quality ones. In

preparation for going to her distributor's store to purchase her new
equipment, Marcia thinks about her various clients and their hair
needs, and makes a list of the new tools she will need to purchase.
Marcia also decides to look for some new styling lotions as well.

88. The foundation tool for all of Marcia's styling begins with
her:
A. styling comb
B. lotions and gels
C. blow-dryer
D. round brush

89. Marcia's blow-dryer must have a/an _____ attachment that
allows the hair to be dried as if it were being air dried.
A. nozzle
B. concentrator
C. diffuser
D. adaptor

90. To detangle wet hair before blow-drying, Marcia will need
to purchase a:
A. fine-toothed comb
B. finger waving comb
C. wide-toothed comb
D. teasing comb

91. For her clients with mid- to longer length hair, Marcia
will need a _____ .
A. classic styling brush
B. paddle brush
C. vent brush
D. large round brush

92. For clients with fine hair or for adding lift at the scalp
area, Marcia will need a:
A. classic styling brush
B. paddle brush
C. vent brush
D. large round brush

93. For clients who need a strong hold styling preparation, Marcia picks up:
    A. styling foam
    B. styling mousse
    C. styling gel
    D. styling pomade

94. For clients who want to add weight to their hair and achieve a piecy, textured look, Marcia purchases:
    A. styling foam
    B. styling mousse
    C. styling gel
    D. styling pomade

95. To add gloss and shine to a finished style, Marcia will need:
    A. hairspray
    B. styling mousse
    C. silicone shiners
    D. styling pomade

THERMAL HAIR STRAIGHTENING

Ternyce has an appointment with Shereen for a shampoo and styling. Ternyce has medium length, layered hair, and she likes to wear it straight, close to the head, and curled under around the face and at the neckline. Ternyce does not chemically straighten her hair.

96. In order for Shereen to style Ternyce's hair, she will need to determine:
    A. how long it is
    B. how much curl to add to it
    C. how clean it is
    D. how much curl to remove from it

97. To remove 100 percent of Ternyce's curl, Shereen will need to use a:
    A. soft press
    B. medium press
    C. hard press
    D. double press

98. Before pressing, Shereen should add ____ to Ternyce's hair and scalp.
    A. pressing dressing
    B. dry shampoo
    C. pressing oil
    D. cholesterol cream

99. To remove 100 percent of Ternyce's curl, and to then curl the hair around the face and under at the nape, Shereen will need to use a:
    A. soft press
    B. medium press
    C. hard press
    D. double press

CHAPTER 13

BRAIDING AND BRAID EXTENSIONS

CLIENT CONSULTATION, UNDERSTANDING THE BASICS, AND BRAIDING THE HAIR

Darshan is interested is having his hair extended through braids and has made an appointment with Lolita for the service. He is told by the receptionist that he will need to be in the salon for several hours so he plans accordingly. Darshan arrives at the salon on time and Lolita begins the service with a client consultation, hair and face analysis, and a discussion about the type and length of the braid and extensions Darshan is looking for. Lolita also takes the time to inform Darshan how to wear and care for his braids before beginning the actual service.

100. Lolita explains that complicated braid styles can last for up to:
    A. 3 days
    B. 30 days
    C. 60 days
    D. 90 days

101. One of the most important aspects of Lolita's client consultation will be to assess the _____ of Darshan's hair.
    A. porosity
    B. elasticity
    C. color
    D. texture

102. Lolita determines that Darshan would look best in a braid style that is full on top and at the neckline, but close to his head at the temples because she has determined that he is a/an _____ facial type.
    A. oval
    B. round
    C. square
    D. diamond

103. In addition to the combs, brushes, and blow-dryer Lolita
     will need for the service, she also sets up her station to
     include the extension materials, _____, and _____.
     A. comb, clips
     B. cape, hackle
     C. drawingboard, hackle
     D. drawingboard, clips

104. Since Darshan intends to wash his hair every two weeks
     and let it dry naturally without the use of heat or irons,
     and he desires a shiny, reflective finished look, the
     material Lolita considers using is:
     A. human hair
     B. kanekalon
     C. nylon
     D. lin

105. Darshan explains that he wants a braid that looks like two
     strands of hair wrapped around one another, called a/an:
     A. inverted braid
     B. rope braid
     C. fishtail braid
     D. extroverted braid

Chapter 14

WIGS AND HAIR ENHANCEMENTS

WIGS

Carlotta has had a number of clients ask her about wigs lately, and she has decided to create a special area within her salon that is dedicated to these items. Clients who are interested in being fitted for a wig or who want to experiment with various wigs will be welcomed to try them out in her salon. Carlotta has several clients who are interested in using the wigs as fashion accessories, so she orders a number of different items from her local distributor.

106. For clients who want the highest quality wigs to cover 100 percent of their hair, Carlotta orders:
    A. synthetic wigs
    B. caplets
    C. human hair wigs
    D. blocks

107. If a client is interested in a product that is ready-to-wear, that comes in fantasy colors, and whose color will not fade, Carlotta should recommend a:
    A. synthetic wig
    B. caplet
    C. human hair wig
    D. block

108. For a client who is interested in an airy type of wig that is less structured, Carlotta should suggest a:
    A. synthetic wig
    B. capless wig
    C. cap wig
    D. block

109. To measure a client for a wig, Carlotta will need a:
    A. hard ruler
    B. block
    C. soft tape measure
    D. weft of hair

110. When customizing the wig to the exact requirements of the client, Carlotta is best able to make alterations to the wig:
    A. on the client's head
    B. on a block
    C. on her own head
    D. on a mannequin

HAIR EXTENSIONS

Judy has had short hair most of her life but has always secretly wanted to try having long hair. But she has difficulty letting her fine, thin hair grow long. She discusses this with her stylist, Linda, who recommends that she consider having a hair extension service. Linda explains that hair extensions come in various forms and amounts and are secured to Judy's existing hair to lengthen the overall style and appearance. Judy books an appointment for the extension service.

111. Before attaching any hair extensions, Linda will need to ascertain from Judy whether or not to:
    A. change her natural hair color
    B. add length to the overall style
    C. tweeze her eyebrows
    D. perm the hair

112. When attaching an extension, it should be placed:
    A. at the front hairline
    B. about three inches from the scalp
    C. just behind the ear
    D. about one inch from the hairline

113. Since Judy has fine hair, Linda will need to:
    A. let her hair grow two inches
    B. give her natural hair a perm
    C. be careful to hide the base of the hair weft
    D. recommend a full wig

114. The best method Linda can use for attaching the hair weft to Linda's fine hair is the _____ method.
    A. track and sew
    B. double-lock stitch
    C. bonding
    D. fusion

Chapter 15

CHEMICAL TEXTURE SERVICES

THE CLIENT CONSULTATION AND PERMANENT WAVING

Mark checks his appointment book and sees that he has three perms scheduled for the day. Anna has short, thick, coarse hair and she is booked for a tight perm so she can wear her hair curly and let it dry naturally. Maureen has medium length, colored hair that is extremely dry. She wants to create additional body in her hair so that it is easier to style and will hold the style a bit longer once she has blown it dry and curled it. And Reva has very long, straight, one-length virgin hair that she is tired of. Instead of cutting the length, Reva wants to try a long and very curly style. To get prepared, Mark stocks his rollabout and retrieves each client's record card.

115. Anna's hair texture indicates to Mark that her hair may:
    A. require less processing time
    B. have too much elasticity
    C. require more processing time
    D. have too little elasticity

116. Since Maureen's hair is colored, Mark must take special care to notice her hair's:
    A. porosity
    B. elasticity
    C. density
    D. texture

117. When wrapping Anna's hair, Mark will employ the ____ technique in order to achieve a tighter curl at the ends and a looser curl at the scalp.
    A. spiral
    B. off-base
    C. croquignole
    D. on-base

118. In order to achieve uniform curl throughout the entire hair strand, Mark will wrap Reva's long hair using the ____ technique.
   A. spiral
   B. off-base
   C. croquignole
   D. on-base

119. To achieve a tighter curl in the center of each strand and a looser curl on the outer edges, Mark will use ____ rods when wrapping Maureen's hair.
   A. round
   B. concave
   C. long
   D. straight

120. To protect the many layers in Maureen's haircut while perming, Mark will employ the ____ wrap.
   A. flat
   B. double flat
   C. single flat
   D. bookend

121. To perm Anna's thick, coarse hair, Mark should select a/an ____ wave.
   A. exothermic
   B. true acid
   C. thio-free
   D. ammonia-free

122. To perm Maureen's extremely damaged hair, Mark should select a/an ____ wave.
   A. exothermic
   B. true acid
   C. thio-free
   D. ammonia-free

123. To perm Reva's virgin hair, Mark should select a/an ____ wave.
   A. cold
   B. true acid
   C. thio-free
   D. ammonia-free

PERMANENT WAVE PROCESSING

Mrs. Carr, who was in the salon two weeks ago for a perm service, has come back into the salon today to tell her stylist Jill that her perm "fried" her hair. She also complains that her hair is curly at the scalp and about halfway down the strand, but the bottom half of the strand is straight, dry, and frizzy. Jill finds Mrs. Carr's record card and reviews the perm she selected and the procedure.

124. Based on Mrs. Carr's description of her hair, her hair is:
    A. underprocessed
    B. neutralized
    C. overprocessed
    D. acidic

125. The perm solution that Jill chose was most likely too:
    A. weak
    B. acidic
    C. strong
    D. neutralized

126. Mrs. Carr's hair doesn't have enough strength left to:
    A. straighten out
    B. remain moisturized
    C. hold the desired curl
    D. grow out naturally

CHEMICAL HAIR RELAXERS AND EXTREMELY CURLY HAIR

Margie has two clients arriving at the salon for appointments. Both Charlotte and Barbara have extremely curly hair that they want to have relaxed. Charlotte wants to wear her hair perfectly straight in a chin length bob style. Barbara wants her hair to be layered, and she wants the curl reduced but not completely taken out so that she can wear her hair wavy. After reviewing their record cards, Maggie realizes that Charlotte had some scalp irritation as a result of her last haircolor appointment. Margie prepares for the services.

127. To completely straighten Charlotte's hair, Margie will use a:
   A. perm wave solution
   B. chemical hair relaxer
   C. soft curl permanent
   D. neutralizer

128. To remove some of the curl from Barbara's hair, Margie will use a:
   A. perm wave solution
   B. chemical hair relaxer
   C. soft curl permanent
   D. neutralizer

129. What should Margie do to determine Charlotte's reaction to the service?
   A. A scalp examination
   B. Use a no-base product
   C. A test curl
   D. Use a protective base

130. A relaxer containing which of the following active ingredient is most appropriate for Margie to use on Charlotte's hair, given her sensitive scalp?
   A. Sodium hydroxide
   B. Lithium hydroxide
   C. Potassium hydroxide
   D. Guanidine hydroxide

131. What strength relaxer is best used on Charlotte?
   A. Mild
   B. Regular
   C. Moderate
   D. Super

132. Barbara's soft curl perm will:
   A. lighten her hair color
   B. make her hair completely straight
   C. reformulate the amount of curl she has
   D. darken her hair color

133. How many services are required for Margie to perform the soft curl perm on Barbara's hair?
    A. 1
    B. 2
    C. 3
    D. 4

134. Which of the following is involved in Margie performing the soft curl perm on Barbara's hair?
    A. Wrapping the hair on perm rods
    B. Relaxing the hair and then recurling it
    C. Relaxing the hair, perming the hair, and rerelaxing the hair
    D. Perming virgin hair, relaxing the hair, and soft curl perming the hair

Chapter 16

HAIRCOLORING

COLOR THEORY

Danny is a master colorist at the Suprema Salon who has a long list of color clients who see him each day. Today, he notices that he has three color correction services planned. The first is Mary who wears light blond highlights and is a swimmer. After swimming in a chlorinated pool every day for the past three months, her hair has a greenish tinge that is unsightly and needs to be corrected. Danny's next client, Amber, colored her own hair at home but was unhappy when her hair turned a brassy orange color. Amber wants to return to her natural color, a deep brown without so much red in it. And Zeena, who recently had her hair bleached from root to ends, wants Danny to change her color because she feels it is too lemony looking.

135. To counteract the greenish tinge in Mary's haircolor, Danny will need to select a shade that has a _____ base color.
    A. blue
    B. yellow
    C. red
    D. violet

136. To prevent Mary's highlighted hair from becoming too dark during the correction procedure, Danny must be careful not to add too much _____ to the color formulation.
    A. blue
    B. yellow
    C. red
    D. violet

137. The color Danny will use to correct Mary's haircolor is a _____ color.
    A. primary
    B. secondary
    C. elementary
    D. tertiary

138. To return Amber's haircolor to the desired shade, Danny will need to use a ____ tone.
    A. warm
    B. brassy
    C. light
    D. cool

139. Typical colors in the tone range Danny will use on Amber's hair have a ____ base.
    A. yellow
    B. orange
    C. red
    D. blue

140. The color Danny will use to correct Amber's brassy tone is a/an ____ color.
    A. duplicate
    B. complementary
    C. tertiary
    D. identical

141. Once achieved, Amber's hair color will be a level:
    A. 10
    B. 7
    C. 5
    D. 3

142. If Zeena wanted her bleached hair to have a cooler, more platinum look instead of the lemony color it is now, Danny will need to select a shade that has a ____ base.
    A. green
    B. yellow
    C. red
    D. violet

143. If Zeena wanted her bleached hair to have a strawberry blond color instead of the lemony color it is now, Danny will need to select a shade that has a ____ base.
    A. green
    B. yellow
    C. red
    D. violet

144. A strawberry blond shade would indicate that Zeena
     preferred a ____ tone in her hair.
     A. warm
     B. brassy
     C. light
     D. cool

145. Once achieved, Zeena's haircolor will be a level:
     A. 10
     B. 7
     C. 5
     D. 3

THE LEVEL SYSTEM AND TYPES OF HAIRCOLOR

Another colorist at the Suprema Salon, Susan, also has a busy day
ahead. She has her first client Gina booked for a color service. Gina has
about 25 percent gray hair and wants something close to her natural
medium brown color to blend and cover her grays. Maya is another of
Susan's clients; she is a natural redhead who wants to have a few
chunky blond highlights around her face. And Katie, who loves to
wear her hair short and funky, and who has been bleaching her hair,
is booked for a full head bleach retouch on a two-inch regrowth area.

146. Since Gina has about 25 percent gray, what is the overall
     situation Susan will encounter when coloring Gina's hair?
     A. Gina has less pigmented hair than gray hair
     B. Gina has more pigmented hair than natural colored
        hair
     C. Gina has more pigmented hair than gray hair
     D. Gina has less pigmented hair than natural colored
        hair

147. To effectively blend Gina's gray hair, Susan should use a:
     A. temporary color
     B. semipermanent color
     C. demipermanent color
     D. permanent color

148. The type of color product Susan uses on Gina should:
    A. add highlights
    B. remove color
    C. deposit color
    D. remove ash tones

149. When formulating Gina's color to ensure proper coverage, Susan should:
    A. select a shade two levels darker than the desired shade
    B. use a shade the desired level straight out of the bottle
    C. mix the color formulation with 40 volume peroxide
    D. select a shade two levels lighter than the desired shade

150. To achieve the chunky highlights that Maya desires, Susan will need to use a/an:
    A. on-the-scalp bleach
    B. cream bleach
    C. oil bleach
    D. off-the-scalp bleach

151. Since Maya's natural hair color is a bright shade of red-orange, her hair will go through _____ degrees of decolorization to achieve the yellow base shade she desires for her highlights.
    A. 3
    B. 4
    C. 5
    D. 6

152. Since Maya has so much red pigment in her hair naturally, Susan may opt to use a _____ technique to achieve a pleasing finished tone to the highlighted hair.
    A. single process coloring
    B. temporary coloring
    C. double process coloring
    D. one-step coloring

153. To lighten Katie's regrowth area, Susan will use a/an:
    A. on-the-scalp bleach
    B. one-step coloring
    C. off-the-scalp bleach
    D. double process coloring

154. To boost the lifting power of the cream bleach, Susan will use a/an:
   A. intimidator
   B. activator
   C. motivator
   D. crystallizer

155. Before applying the toner to Katie's hair, Susan may choose to use a/an_____ to protect and condition the previously bleached hair.
   A. activator
   B. color filler
   C. booster
   D. conditioner filler

156. After her hair is lightened to the desired level, Susan should formulate and tone Katie's hair using a ____ volume developer to simply add color and lessen the amount of damage done to the hair.
   A. 10
   B. 20
   C. 30
   D. 40

157. Which of Susan's clients requires a patch test before she begins their services?
   A. None of them
   B. Maya only
   C. Gina only
   D. All of them

Part IV—SKIN CARE

Chapter 17

HISTOLOGY OF THE SKIN

ANATOMY OF THE SKIN

Clare has returned from a week-long vacation in the Bahamas and has made an appointment with Donna, an esthetician, for a facial. While examining her skin, Donna notices that Clare has a tan, and that in certain areas on her face and neck, the skin is taut, pink, dry, and painful to the touch. Clare complains that she is beginning to see wrinkles around her mouth and eyes, that the skin on her nose is a bit oily, and there are dark spots imbedded in the skin.

1. During her examination, Donna is observing Clare's:
   A. epidermis
   B. papillary layer
   C. dermis
   D. reticular layer

2. Clare's tan is a result of the effect of ultraviolet rays that increased the amount of ____ in her skin.
   A. keratin
   B. stratum lucidum
   C. melanin
   D. stratum granulosum

3. The appearance of skin that is taut, pink, and dry indicates that Clare may have a:
   A. tan
   B. SPF
   C. sunburn
   D. nerve disorder

4. What is causing Clare's wrinkles?
   A. Laughing too much
   B. Loss of collagen and elastin
   C. Not squinting enough
   D. Too much collagen and elastin

5. Which nerves are responsible for the pain Clare feels?
   A. Motor nerve fibers
   B. Sensory nerve fibers
   C. Elastin nerve fibers
   D. Secretory nerve fibers

6. Which nerves are responsible for Clare's nose being oily?
   A. Motor nerve fibers
   B. Sensory nerve fibers
   C. Elastin nerve fibers
   D. Secretory nerve fibers

7. The nerves that are responsible for Clare's nose being oily
   are located in the _____ of the skin.
   A. stratum lucidum
   B. epidermis
   C. reticular layer
   D. stratum corneum

8. The dark spots that are imbedded in the skin on Clare's
   nose are called:
   A. milia
   B. comedones
   C. seborrhea
   D. rosacea

9. These dark spots are caused by:
   A. hardened sebum in a hair follicle
   B. discoloration of the cells
   C. the accumulation of dry skin
   D. loosened debris

10. These dark spots are considered to be a disorder of the:
    A. sweat glands
    B. sudoriferous glands
    C. sebacceous glands
    D. mammary glands

DISORDERS OF THE SKIN

Gigi is a runner who has just completed a five-mile marathon. She has just come across the finish line and is drenched in perspiration and breathing heavily. This was a difficult race for Gigi because it was a very hot day with high humidity, and as a result of running through a wooded area, she has several mosquito bites on her arms and legs, which she had been scratching as often as she could while running. Also, under her arms, Gigi notices a mass of small reds bumps that burn when she moves her arms back and forth. After a few moments, Gigi takes off her running shoes and notices a foul smell.

11. Gigi's perspiration is a function of the:
    A. sebaceous glands
    B. motor nerve fibers
    C. sweat glands
    D. sensory nerve fibers

12. The itchy, swollen lesion caused by Gigi's mosquito bite is called a:
    A. cyst
    B. pustule
    C. vesicle
    D. wheal

13. While running, the sweat glands in Clare's ____ make adjustments to allow her to be cooled by the evaporation of sweat.
    A. sebaceous glands
    B. skin
    C. oil glands
    D. fundus

14. To protect herself from overexposure to the sun while running, Gigi should have worn a:
    A. wide brimmed hat
    B. capri pants
    C. sunscreen
    D. baseball cap

15. As a result of scratching the mosquito bites on her arms, Gigi had developed a/an:
    A. crust
    B. excoriation
    C. fissure
    D. keloid

16. The mass of small reds bumps that burn when Gigi moves her arms back and forth are called:
    A. eczema
    B. anhidrosis
    C. milaria rubra
    D. bromhidrosis

17. The foul odor Gigi notices after removing her running shoes is called:
    A. eczema
    B. anhidrosis
    C. milaria rubra
    D. bromhidrosis

Dr. Tinsley is a dermatologist who sees patients with all sorts of skin disorders. Today, she has several patients waiting to see her. Brent is a construction worker who works in many types of weather conditions. His hands have a tremendous amount of hard, dried skin on them that sometimes cracks and becomes painful. Pam has developed a dark colored, red wine spot on her forehead that only started to appear after a long illness she recently overcame. Mrs. Fagan has noticed a number of small, light brown colored outgrowths of skin on her neck and wants to make sure they are not harmful to her health. Maryann has a large, dark, raised spot on her chest and has recently noticed a hair growing out of it, and decided to check in with the doctor about it.

18. Brent's hands contain:
    A. stains
    B. skin tags
    C. calluses
    D. moles

19. Pam's discolored spot is called a:
    A. stain
    B. skin tag
    C. callus
    D. mole

20. What caused the discolored spot on Pam's forehead?
    A. Overexposure to the sun
    B. Certain medications
    C. There is no known cause
    D. Too many trips to the tanning bed

21. Mrs. Fagan's outgrowths of skin are called:
    A. stains
    B. skin tags
    C. calluses
    D. moles

22. When do these outgrowths normally appear?
    A. When a person changes jobs
    B. When a person ages
    C. When a person moves to a warmer climate
    D. When a person colors her hair

23. What is the dark colored spot on Maryanne's chest?
    A. A carbuncle
    B. A comedone
    C. A mole
    D. A tumor

Chapter 18

HAIR REMOVAL

CLIENT CONSULTATION, AND PERMANENT AND TEMPORARY METHODS OF HAIR REMOVAL

Joanie is a fashion conscience businesswoman who deals with the public all day long. She is very careful to present a professional and attractive appearance. Joanie has always had a problem with superfluous facial and body hair. Once a week, she shapes her eyebrows at home with a pair of tweezers, and every other week, when she has her nails done, she also books an appointment for removal of unsightly facial hair on her upper lip, chin, and neck. Joanie undergoes waxing although sometimes it irritates her face. Joanie usually shaves the hair on her legs and underarms every other day but her skin often feels bumpy from shaving so often. Joanie wants to investigate some other options for hair removal that may make her personal grooming routine easier and less bothersome. She discusses her options with Amber, her esthetician.

24. Before determining the appropriate methods of hair removal, a positive answer to which of the following questions would indicate to Amber that she should not be providing hair removal services for Joanie?
    A. Do you suffer from oily skin patches?
    B. Have you ever had a mud mask?
    C. Do you currently use Retin-A?
    D. Are you a frequent tanning salon client?

25. When Joanie shapes her own eyebrows with the pair of tweezers, she is using a method called:
    A. permanent hair removal
    B. photoepilation
    C. sugaring
    D. temporary hair removal

26. If Amber was to discuss methods of permanent hair removal with Joanie, she would suggest:
    A. electrolysis, tweezing, and epilation
    B. photoepilation, shaving, and depilatories
    C. laser hair removal, electronic tweezers, and waxing
    D. electrolysis, photoepilation, and laser hair removal

27. A quick and easy method of temporary hair removal Amber could suggest for removing the hair on Joanie's legs that would not leave the skin smooth but requires a patch test is:
    A. a depilatory
    B. photoepilation
    C. sugaring
    D. tweezing

28. A milder but equally effective way of removing Joanie's facial hair could be to:
    A. wax
    B. tweeze
    C. shave
    D. sugar

29. To minimize the irritation to Joanie's underarms, Amber suggests the use of:
    A. hot wax
    B. shaving
    C. depilatories
    D. cold wax

Chapter 19

FACIALS

BASIC CLASSIFICATION AND CHEMISTRY OF SKIN CARE PRODUCTS

Rebecca, an esthetician, is asked by a high school counselor to visit a class of graduating students to discuss skin care with them. She arrives with product samples and begins to explain about the skin, its function, and how best to care for it. When she opens the floor to questions, she receives many questions from three students—Jane, Anne, and Andrea—about types and uses of skin care products available on the market and how best to use them. Rebecca is happy to answer the questions and reduce confusion.

30. Anne asks Rebecca about the difference between a face wash and a cleansing cream. Rebecca tells her that:
    A. a face wash removes makeup; a cleansing cream does not.
    B. a cleansing cream is usually best used on very oily skin
    C. a face wash is not useful for people with acne
    D. a face wash is a detergent-like foaming cleanser; a cleansing cream dissolves makeup quickly

31. Jane explains that she has some acne and asks what she should use to cleanse her face. Rebecca suggests a:
    A. bar of soap
    B. face wash
    C. cleansing cream
    D. cleansing lotion

32. For Andrea's dry and sensitive skin, Rebecca recommends using a/an ____ after cleansing.
    A. alcohol
    B. tonic
    C. freshener
    D. astringent

33. Jane complains that her skin appears bumpy and lumpy. Rebecca recommends that she use a/an ____ two to three times a week.
    A. cleansing cream
    B. tonic
    C. astringent
    D. exfoliant

34. Andrea tells Rebecca that her facialist suggested an enzyme peel but that she wasn't sure what it was. Rebecca responded by explaining that it is a/an:
    A. exfoliating procedure using fruit acids
    B. cleansing procedure using banana peels
    C. acne treatment using a nourishing cream
    D. exfoliating procedure using keratolytic enzymes

35. Jane asks Rebecca if there is anything she can use on her skin daily to reduce dryness. Rebecca suggests a:
    A. massage cream
    B. night cream
    C. moisturizer
    D. treatment cream

36. Andrea wonders if there is any special treatment that can be useful on oily skin. Rebecca explains that a ____ mask will help reduce sebum production.
    A. clay
    B. paraffin
    C. sulfur
    D. modelage

FACIAL MASSAGE

Patricia has booked a facial at her favorite salon and can't wait for the soothing massage to begin. She arrives, changes into a facial gown, and waits patiently for her esthetician, Alma, to arrive. The lights are dim and there is soft music playing in the background. Before entering the room Alma reviews Patricia's client record card and notices that the last time she was in, she commented that she wanted to tone her muscles and improve her circulation and general health. Alma enters the room and begins the service.

37. Alma begins by using a technique that involves a light, continuous, stroking movement called:
    A. petrissage
    B. effleurage
    C. fulling
    D. chucking

38. To offer deep stimulation to Patricia's muscles, Alma employs:
    A. petrissage
    B. effleurage
    C. friction
    D. chucking

39. To increase Patricia's circulation and glandular activity, Alma uses a ____ technique.
    A. petrissage
    B. effleurage
    C. friction
    D. chucking

40. Alma uses ____ on Patricia's neck to tone her muscles.
    A. wringing
    B. effleurage
    C. tapotement
    D. chucking

41. Alma is always careful to massage from the:
    A. origin to the outset
    B. outset to the inset
    C. insertion to the origin
    D. origin to the insertion

ELECTROTHERAPY AND LIGHT THERAPY

Albert sells electric facial machines to salons that help enhance the effectiveness of facial treatments. He has a meeting with Joyce to review her needs for additional equipment and special appliances. When Albert arrives, Joyce is ready and waiting for him with a list of questions.

42. Joyce asks if there is any electrotherapy treatment that will help liquefy sebum on the face of a client. Albert explains that the application of ____ will do just that.
    A. galvanic current
    B. faradic current
    C. sinusoidal current
    D. high-frequency current

43. To tone the facial muscles of older clients, Joyce is interested in using:
    A. galvanic current
    B. light therapy
    C. faradic current
    D. high-frequency current

44. For use on acne-prone skin, Albert explains the use of ____ will help the skin accept the treatment more deeply.
    A. galvanic current
    B. light therapy
    C. faradic current
    D. high-frequency current

Paulette offers a variety of light therapies in her skin care salon and has a private room with a therapeutic lamp for these treatments. Paulette notes that several of her clients will benefit from the light therapies: Mark, who fell two weeks ago and is having back pain; Michelle, who is being plagued by skin eruptions; Allie, the computer programmer, whose shoulders and neck always hurt her; Amy, who loves to have tanned skin but is careful not to expose herself to the sun; and Mrs. Halperin, whose skin is very dry and wrinkled.

45. To soothe Mark's aching back, Paulette will place him under a/an ____ light.
    A. blue
    B. infrared
    C. white
    D. ultraviolet

46. To educe Michelle's skin eruptions, Paulette will place her under a/an ____ light.
    A. blue
    B. infrared
    C. white
    D. ultraviolet

47. To alleviate Allie's sore shoulders and neck, Paulette will place her under a/an ____ light.
    A. blue
    B. infrared
    C. white
    D. ultraviolet

48. Amy will tan under a ____ light.
    A. red
    B. infrared
    C. white
    D. ultraviolet

49. To reduce the appearance of Mrs. Halperin's dry and wrinkled skin, Paulette will use a ____ light.
    A. red
    B. infrared
    C. white
    D. ultraviolet

Chapter 20

FACIAL MAKEUP

COSMETICS FOR FACIAL MAKEUP

Amanda has booked a makeup appointment with Sandra for the morning of her wedding. She has discussed the color of her wedding gown—off-white—and her belief that she looks best in orange or coral tones with Sandra. Sandra notes that Amanda has deep auburn colored hair, light pale skin, and large green colored eyes. The morning of her wedding, Amanda arrives at the salon with a freshly cleansed, toned, and moisturized face, but she has a blemish on her forehead and some dark circles under her eyes. Sandra starts the application.

50. From the information that Sandra has received about Amanda's color preferences and from analyzing her skin, she determines that her skin tone is:
    A. cool
    B. cold
    C. hot
    D. warm

51. Before any other product goes on Amanda's face, and to even out her skin tone and create a base for the makeup application, Sandra applies:
    A. concealor
    B. foundation
    C. face powder
    D. cheek color

52. To cover Amanda's blemish and to reduce the discoloration around her eyes, Sandra will apply a concealor whose color is:
    A. lighter than the skin tone
    B. the same as the skin tone
    C. heavier than the skin tone
    D. darker than the skin tone

53. To set the foundation, concealor, and to give the face a matte finish, Sandra pats on a:
    A. concealor
    B. foundation
    C. face powder
    D. cheek color

54. To keep her makeup matte-looking, Sandra adds ____ cheek color.
    A. gel
    B. cream
    C. dry
    D. liquid

55. To harmonize with Amanda's coloring, she should wear a ____ color on her cheeks.
    A. pink
    B. mauve
    C. coral
    D. burgundy

56. To keep Amanda's lip color from feathering, Sandra applies:
    A. lip color
    B. concealor
    C. foundation
    D. lip liner

57. Sandra fills in Amanda's lips with:
    A. lip color
    B. concealor
    C. foundation
    D. lip liner

58. The best lip color to apply is:
    A. warm toned
    B. blue-red
    C. cool toned
    D. light pink

59. To make Amanda's green eyes a focal point, Sandra should select a _____ color.
    A. deep blue
    B. silver grey
    C. plum
    D. green

60. Sandra highlights Amanda's eyes with a color that is:
    A. lighter than the skin tone
    B. the same as the skin tone
    C. heavier than the skin tone
    D. darker than the skin tone

61. To make Amanda's eyes appear larger and more open, Sandra should apply:
    A. eyeliner across the top
    B. mascara on the top lashes only
    C. eye color in the crease
    D. mascara on top and bottom lashes

CORRECTIVE MAKEUP

Linda is a makeup artist who works for a high-end cosmetics line sold exclusively through salons and spas. Today, a distributor is hosting an educational conference where Linda will be the guest speaker. The topic of today's class will be corrective makeup techniques and Linda will be demonstrating these techniques using the cosmetics line she represents. Instead of hiring models, the conference participants will analyze and perform the corrective techniques on one another. Courtney, one of the class participants, is first. She has a wide forehead and cheek area but a rather narrow jawline, small eyes, and a very long, thin neck. Carmen, another participant, has a very full, round face, with a wide and some-what flat nose, protruding eyes, and a rather thick chin and neck area. Rita has a very low forehead and a thin upper lip.

62. What face shape does Courtney have?
    A. Diamond
    B. Triangle
    C. Square
    D. Inverted triangle

63. To make Courtney's face appear more oval, Linda will need to:
   A. offset the hard edges at the chin and jawline
   B. minimize the width of the forehead and increase the width of the jawline
   C. create width at the forehead and slenderize the jawline
   D. create the illusion of a wider check bone area

64. To make Courtney's small eyes appear larger, Linda will:
   A. apply shadow to the outer corners of the eye only
   B. apply shadow in the crease
   C. blend the eye shadow over the upper lid
   D. extend the eye shadow above, beyond, and below the eye

65. To create more fullness to Courtney's neck and jawline area, Linda decides to apply a _____ to the area.
   A. dark concealor
   B. translucent powder
   C. light foundation
   D. bronzing lotion

66. To make Carmen's round face appear slimmer, she will need to:
   A. offset the hard edges at the chin and jawline
   B. create width at the forehead and slenderize the jawline
   C. create the illusion of a wider check bone area
   D. slenderize and lengthen the face

67. To correct Carmen's wide, flat nose, Linda will:
   A. apply a light foundation on either side of the nostrils
   B. apply a line of extra light foundation down the center of the nose
   C. apply a dark foundation on either side of the nostrils
   D. apply a line of extra dark foundation down the center of the nose

68. To minimize her protruding eyes, Carmen should:
    A. use a light, pearly color on the entire eye lid
    B. blend a deep shade of shadow over the upper lid and to the eyebrow
    C. use a highlight color in the crease and upper eyelid
    D. use a medium toned shadow at the crease line

69. To slenderize Carmen's neck and jawline area, Linda will apply a ____ to the area.
    A. dark foundation
    B. translucent powder
    C. light foundation
    D. bronzing lotion

70. To give the appearance of a more balanced face, Rita can offset her low forehead with eyebrows that have a:
    A. high arch
    B. medium arch
    C. low arch
    D. no arch

71. How can Linda correct Rita's thin upper lip?
    A. by using a dark color on the upper and lower lips
    B. by using a lip pencil to make the curve of the bottom lip proportionate to the chin
    C. by using a lip pencil to make the curves of the upper lips proportionate to the nostrils
    D. by using a light, frosted shade on the upper and lower lips

Part V—NAIL CARE

Chapter 21

NAIL STRUCTURE AND GROWTH

NAIL GROWTH AND NAIL DISORDERS

Ellie has been a nail technician for more than 20 years, and in the course of her career, she has had many clients with nail disorders and problems that can be serviced and helped through regular nail care and maintenance.

1. While recovering from a serious heart attack, Mrs. Jones' nails developed wavy ridges. Ellie recognized the condition as:
   A. blue nail
   B. corrugations
   C. hangnail
   D. onychophagy

2. Ruben gave his daughter a gift certificate for a manicure with Ellie in the hopes that it would arrest her onychophagy, a condition where she _____ her nails.
   A. paints
   B. cuts
   C. bites
   D. pulls out

3. After losing more than 100 pounds on a fad diet, Sabrina noticed that her nails were noticeably thinner, whiter, and more flexible than normal; Ellie explained that this is called _____.
   A. blue nail
   B. eggshell nails
   C. hangnail
   D. pterygium

4. Raul has very thick nails that seem to grow in layers. He has:
   A. hangnail
   B. pterygium
   C. onychauxis
   D. onychatrophia

5. After Sabrina slammed her hand into the table when she fell at home, she noticed a whitish discoloration of her nails. Ellie told her this was called ____ and caused by injury to the base of the nail.
   A. pterygium
   B. plicatured nails
   C. leukonchia
   D. melanonychia

Wendy, a loyal acrylic nail wearer, has been going to Cecilia for more than three years. Recently, she noticed a dark greenish spot appear on her index finger nail. At first she ignored it, but over time, it became darker, and eventually she noticed that it had a foul odor.

6. What is the green spot?
   A. A mold
   B. A bacterial infection
   C. An old nail tip
   D. Dirt

7. The green spot is most likely caused by:
   A. using acetone that was too strong for the nail polish
   B. trapped moisture between the natural nail and the enhancement
   C. cutting the natural nail too frequently
   D. wearing an enhancement that is longer than 1/4 inch

8. How will this nail most likely be cured?
   A. By cutting it off at the free edge
   B. By cleansing it with warm sudsy water
   C. By exposing it to air
   D. By painting over it with a dark polish

NAIL DISEASES

Raul attends a nail care seminar, and one of the classes is conducted by Dr. Reddy, a medical doctor, who is discussing the types of nail diseases a nail technician should be aware of. He uses a slide projector with photographic examples of each kind of disease he discusses.

9. The first slide Dr. Reddy shows is of a nail that is separated from and falling off of the nail bed. This condition is called:
    A. onychia
    B. oncholysis
    C. onchomadesis
    D. onchoptosis

10. The next slide depicts a nail with an inflamed matrix with pus and shedding. This condition is called:
    A. onychia
    B. oncholysis
    C. onchomadesis
    D. onchoptosis

11. Dr. Reddy shows another slide and explains that growth of horny epithelium in the nail bed is called:
    A. onychia
    B. oncholysis
    C. onchomadesis
    D. onchophosis

12. Dr. Reddy's next slide is of a man's foot with what appear to be deep, itchy, colorless blisters. These are:
    A. athlete's foot
    B. clubbed foot
    C. hammer toes
    D. stubbed toes

Chapter 22

MANICURING AND PEDICURING

NAIL CARE TOOLS

Josie is a new nail technician at the Helpful Hands Nail Salon. On her first day, she sets up her manicure station with all of her tools and implements and gets ready for her first client, Wanda. Wanda arrives and requests a natural nail manicure and hands Josie a bottle of bright red nail polish she has brought into the salon with her. Josie gets to work.

13. The first thing that Josie does is:
    A. file the nails
    B. cut the cuticle
    C. remove the old nail polish
    D. place the hands into the finger bowl

14. To shape Wanda's nails, Josie will use a/an:
    A. cuticle nipper
    B. orangewood stick
    C. cotton pledglet
    D. emery board

15. Wanda explains that she would like her nails shorter, so Josie uses a ____ to shorten them to the desired length.
    A. nail buffer
    B. cuticle nipper
    C. orangewood stick
    D. nail clipper

16. Josie recommends that Wanda consider using a ____ daily to correct and prevent brittle nails and dry cuticles.
    A. cuticle oil
    B. base coat
    C. cuticle cream
    D. dry nail polish

17. Before applying the polish and base coat, Josie applies a
    ____ to strengthen the nails and prevent them from
    splitting or peeling.
    A. nail color
    B. cuticle cream
    C. nail dryer
    D. nail hardener

18. How should Josie remove excess nail polish from around
    Wanda's nails?
    A. By removing all of the polish and painting the nail
       again
    B. With a cotton-tipped orangewood stick dipped in
       polish remover
    C. By spraying nail dryer on the nail, then removing all
       of the polish from the nail
    D. With a cotton pledglet while the nail polish is still
       wet.

PEDICURES

Jose is a retail store manager who spends hundreds of hours a month
on his feet. For his birthday, his wife Leona has booked an appointment for him to have a pedicure with Joya, a pedicurist at their local
salon. When he arrives for the appointment, he explains to Joya that
he is eager to have his feet massaged. Joya begins the service.

19. Before getting to the foot massage, Joya must:
    A. remove toenail polish, apply toe separators, and trim
       the toenails
    B. clip and file toenails, file down rough skin, and place
       the feet in the foot bath
    C. soak feet in the foot bath, remove polish, and file the
       feet with a nail rasp
    D. insert toe separators, soak the feet in the foot bath,
       and clip the toenails

20. To push back the cuticle and finish the pedicure, Joya will use a:
    A. liquid soap and a cotton-tipped orangewood stick
    B. foot lotion and a nail rasp
    C. a diamond nail file and cuticle cream
    D. cuticle solvent and a cotton-tipped orangewood stick

21. Once the pedicure is completed, Joya will begin the massage with the ____ technique for relation.
    A. thumb compression
    B. percussion
    C. effleurage
    D. metatarsal scissors

22. Next, Joya will move on to a ____ massage technique, which will promote flexibility and stimulate blood flow.
    A. thumb compression
    B. percussion
    C. effleurage
    D. metatarsal scissors

23. To further stimulate blood flow, Joya will use the ____ technique.
    A. thumb compression
    B. percussion
    C. fist twist
    D. metatarsal scissors

24. Joya will end the massage with a technique called ____ to reduce the blood flow.
    A. thumb compression
    B. percussion
    C. fist twist
    D. metatarsal scissors

DISINFECTING FOOT SPAS

Please refer to Chapter 5, Infection Control, page 115 in *Milady's Standard Cosmetology*, 2004 ed.

Heather has just hired a new pedicurist, Allie, who has finished her training and is eager to start work at her very first salon job.

Heather gives Allie a quick tour of the salon, then instructs Allie on where the salon's disinfectants are stored and on how to disinfect the foot spas that are used for pedicure clients, including instructions on how and when to clean and disinfect the foot baths.

25. Heather instructs Allie to ____ after draining the water and removing foreign matter from the foot spa after each client.
    A. store the foot bath in a dark cool place
    B. clean the surfaces and walls with soap and water
    C. dry the foot bath with a clean towel
    D. spray the foot bath with alcohol

26. Next, Heather explains that Allie will need to disinfect the foot bath with a/an ____ disinfectant, according to the manufacturers' directions.
    A. NCA-registered
    B. FDA-registered
    C. EPA-registered
    D. ANC-registered

27. At the end of each day, Heather tells Allie that she will need to:
    A. add a cup of bleach to the water and leave the foot bath running for two hours
    B. circulate alcohol through the foot bath for 5 to 10 minutes
    C. spray a foot deodorizer into the foot bath and allow it to dry completely
    D. remove the screen and clean the debris trapped behind it

28. When washing the screen and inlet, Allie may use a ____ percent chlorine solution.
    A. 5
    B. 15
    C. 25
    D. 50

29. To flush the system at the end of the day, Allie should use a low-sudsing soap and warm water, and allow it to filter through the system for:
    A. one hour
    B. 15 minutes
    C. 10 minutes
    D. one day

30. Heather tells Allie that every two weeks she will need to fill the foot spa tub with water and four teaspoons of 5 percent bleach solution and let the solution sit:
    A. for two days
    B. an hour
    C. overnight
    D. for five minutes

CHAPTER 23

ADVANCED NAIL TECHNIQUES

NAIL WRAPS

Roberta has been a nail technician for many years and has a thriving clientele. While many of the nail salons in her area tend to specialize in one type of nail enhancement, Roberta is adept at performing and servicing every type of nail service a client may require. Today, she will be seeing several clients who each require a different type of nail service. Kelly, her first client, is new to the salon, and is scheduled for tips and wraps. Her second client, Joanne, wears acrylic nails; and her third client, Nicole, wears gel nails.

31. In order to determine the best type of wrap for Kelly, Roberta will need to ask her which of the following questions?
    A. What color polishes do you most like to wear?
    B. Do you plan on having nail art over the finished nails?
    C. How rough are you on your hands and nails?
    D. Would you like to have a pedicure while you are here?

32. Kelly explains that she is a landscape artist, and she works outdoors planning and gardening all day long. Based on this, Roberta recommends that she wear ____ wraps for durability.
    A. silk
    B. fiberglass
    C. linen
    D. paper

33. Kelly asks Roberta about maintaining her new nails. Roberta explains that her nails must be:
    A. manicured every two weeks
    B. glued every two weeks and rewrapped every four weeks
    C. rewrapped every two weeks
    D. rewrapped every two weeks and glued every four weeks

34. Joanne wears nail tips with acrylic overlays, so when Roberta does Joanne's nails, she uses:
    A. nail forms and primer
    B. a monomer and polymer
    C. a monomer and nail form
    D. a catalyst and nail tips

35. To aid in the adhesion and to prepare the nail surface for attachment with the acrylic material, Roberta will use _____ on Joanne's' nails.
    A. monomer
    B. polymer
    C. catalyst
    D. primer

36. Once applied, acrylic overlays should be _____ every two weeks and the shape of the nail should be _____ each time acrylic is used.
    A. refilled, balanced
    B. filled, changed
    C. refilled, cut
    D. filled, balanced

37. The completion of Nicole's gel nail application will require Roberta to use two steps: _____ and _____.
    A. application, removal
    B. lighting, hardening
    C. application, hardening
    D. lightening, removal

38. Roberta chooses a no-light gel for Nicole's nails, so she may need to _____ to finish the nail application.
    A. spray nail dryer on the nails
    B. put Nicole's nails into an oil bath
    C. immerse Nicole's hands in water
    D. massage Nicole's arms and elbows

Part VI—THE BUSINESS OF COSMETOLOGY

Chapter 24

THE SALON BUSINESS

GOING INTO BUSINESS FOR YOURSELF

Don has been a stylist for more than six years and has built a loyal clientele at his current salon. He has thought about moving out and opening his own salon for several months and has decided to explore all the various options open to him. He calls his friends—Emily, Scott, and Matt—who are stylists at different salons in the area and they agree to get together after work to discuss options and share ideas with Don.

1. Emily tells Don that she is a _____, which means that she pays rent to a salon owner for the space she works in, supplies all of her own materials and products, and has complete control over her work schedule and appointments.
   A. partner
   B. coowner
   C. booth renter
   D. sole proprietor

2. Scott is a _____ of the Scott Salon and is responsible for determining all the policies of the salon, hiring and paying all the employees, and he assumes all the responsibilities of the expenses and profits of the salon.
   A. partner
   B. coowner
   C. booth renter
   D. sole proprietor

3. Matt explains that he is a ____ with his wife, Anne. They share all of the duties of owning the business and all of the rewards as well. Since he is a cosmetologist, he manages the salon while his wife, who is an accountant, manages the finances and operations.
   A. partner
   B. coowner
   C. booth renter
   D. sole proprietor

4. Scott advises Don to be aware of the area in which he will be working. He explains that ____, ____, ____, and ____ are important factors in determining where to open a new salon and whether or not it will be successful.
   A. color palette, decor, furniture, draperies
   B. demographics, visibility, parking, competition
   C. style magazines, hair posters, reception literature, retail stations
   D. cutting tools, rollabouts, mirrors, styling implements

5. Don's friends advise him to develop a ____, which will help him clarify his vision and determine which type of opportunity is best for him.
   A. job description
   B. business plan
   C. will
   D. letter of resignation

After careful consideration, Don has decided to open his own salon as a sole proprietorship. He writes an extensive business plan outlining his vision for his business, and creates a budget to determine what his expenses will and should be. Don takes his business plan and budget to his local bank and meets with John Burke, the small business loan officer, to see about getting a loan to open his new salon.

6. John asks Don how much ____ he is seeking to run the salon for the first two years.
   A. space
   B. investment
   C. capital
   D. interest

7. John asks Don what percentage of the overall salon revenue he expects to spend on rent for the space and for advertising.
   A. Approximately 3%
   B. Approximately 13%
   C. Approximately 16%
   D. Approximately 26%

8. To make informed decisions about the salon's financial success, Don explains to John that he will keep ____ and ____ records to control expenses and waste.
   A. hourly, daily
   B. daily, weekly
   C. hourly, weekly
   D. weekly, monthly

9. Don mentions that ____ supplies such as hairspray and styling products will be on hand to sell to salon clients so that they can maintain their styles at home and that these sales will increase the salon's profitability.
   A. consumption
   B. back room
   C. service
   D. retail

10. John asks to see a copy of the projected ____ so that he can asses whether or not the salon will have the correct flow, and be conducive to the many services and the demands of the clients who will patronize it.
    A. newspaper ads
    B. service menu
    C. salon layout
    D. price list

OPERATING A SUCCESSFUL SALON AND MANAGING PERSONNEL

Andrew is the manager at the Peaceful Mind Salon and Spa, a luxurious day spa that caters to many wealthy clients. He has just been to a manager's meeting with the salon's owners and has learned that in three months, the salon will need to move to another location, and when they do, there will be some management and operational changes introduced. He realizes that this will be very disruptive to the salon clients and to the personnel who have worked at the salon for a long time, and who have well-established clients and are making a comfortable living because of the loyal client base. Andrew has a staff meeting with his salon staff in two days and he has to decide whether or not to discuss the salon move and all of the changes it will bring.

11. As the salon manager, and to help his staff ease into the move, Andrew should:
    A. delay telling the staff until they have to actually pack their stations for the move
    B. be honest about the situation and provide updates when they are available
    C. allude that there may be a move in store but not give any details
    D. tell them that he heard a rumor that there may be some big changes coming

12. Since Andrew knows that once the move is announced, some of his longtime staffers may experience feelings of uncertainty and fear, he offers to:
    A. find them new jobs
    B. oppose the move to the owners
    C. listen and help them with their issues
    D. help them get copies of their client lists so they can leave

13. For those decisions that he can share with his staff, and for those issues that can be resolved by the staff, Andrew should consider:
    A. making the decision and simply relaying that information to the staff
    B. sharing the decision-making with the staff when it is feasible to do so
    C. asking the salon's owners to make the decision on how to resolve the problem
    D. looking at how other salons solve a similar problem and simply adapting their resolution

THE FRONT DESK

Marta is the receptionist at the Intrigue Salon and she handles more than 40 salon guests per day. The salon has a large reception area that is home to the more than 10 retail lines of products the salon sells, as well as the central location for all clients to fill in paperwork and wait for their appointments. Marta is also responsible for answering all of the phone calls that come into the salon on three phone lines and for booking appointments for salon guests. On this particular day, Marta is handling a very demanding client who is upset because she is being kept waiting for her haircut appointment. In the midst of trying to help the client, the telephone rings.

14. Marta should:
    A. ignore the phone and continue trying to help the upset client
    B. yell to one of the stylist to pick up the phone
    C. excuse herself briefly from the client and answer the call
    D. reach over and pick up the phone as a means of getting away from the upset client

15. If Marta chooses to answer the call and help the caller, how should she resume her conversation with the upset client?
    A. By ignoring her complaints and offering her a cup of coffee
    B. By determining when the stylist can begin her service and offering to reschedule her appointment if she prefers
    C. By pulling the late stylist aside and telling her to deal with the unhappy client
    D. By creating a complicated reason why the stylist is late and explaining that if she just sits down, she'll be next

16. If Marta chooses not to answer the call, she may be missing an important opportunity for the salon to:
    A. seek new employment
    B. change an appointment for a client
    C. speak to her boyfriend
    D. buy a product from a telemarketer's offer

17. To make the upset client happy and to keep her as a salon regular, Marta should:

A. tell her that the service will be free

B. gossip about how her stylist is always late, which puts her behind schedule every day

C. make an appointment for her at another salon for the same day

D. ask how she would like to remedy the problem and get approval from salon management

Chapter 25

SEEKING EMPLOYMENT

PREPARING FOR LICENSURE AND THE TEST, AND DEDUCTIVE REASONING

Samuel has just received a notice from his state board of cosmetology that he is scheduled to take his licensing exam in two weeks. He is happy but also nervous about taking the exam, and he wants very badly to pass the test on his first try. But he always has had trouble taking examinations because of his nerves. Samuel pulls out his textbook and study materials, and begins to schedule his study and preparation time.

18. Samuel should begin studying:
     A. the day before the test
     B. the evening before the exam
     C. the morning of the exam
     D. several weeks before the exam

19. In order to get ready for his written exam, Samuel should:
     A. practice his finger waving technique
     B. take time to party with his buddies right before the exam
     C. have a drink the morning of the exam to help him relax
     D. review past quizzes, tests, and homework assignments

20. The evening before the exam, Samuel should plan to:
     A. study all night long
     B. get about four hours sleep
     C. go out and forget about the exam
     D. get a full night's sleep

21. Once he is given the exam, Samuel should:
    A. begin answering the questions in the order they are presented
    B. answer all the questions by marking A next to each
    C. read through the exam and all of the directions before beginning the test
    D. answer all the questions by marking C next to each

22. If Samuel is stuck on a question, he can _____ and then determine which are possible correct answers.
    A. skip to a question he can answer
    B. eliminate answers he knows are incorrect
    C. look at another person's sheet
    D. opt to take only the practical exam

PREPARING FOR EMPLOYMENT

Amira has graduated from beauty school, received passing grades on her exams, and wants to find a good salon job. She begins looking in various local newspapers for job openings and makes a list of salons that have openings. She makes several appointments with many of the salons who ran ads in the newspaper to apply for their open positions. She dresses well in an outfit with matching shoes and handbag, has her hair and makeup done beautifully, and has had her car washed so that she presents a great-looking appearance to her prospective salon manager.

23. When she arrives at the first salon, the manager asks Amira for her credentials. She should hand her a:
    A. photo of herself doing hair
    B. resume
    C. reference letter
    D. business card

24. What kinds of information will the manager need to ascertain about Amira before determining if she is right for the open position?
    A. Her marital status
    B. Her job history
    C. Her product preferences
    D. Her favorite clothing designer

25. Another tool Amira should consider taking with her on interviews is a/an:
    A. photo album of hairstyles from popular magazines
    B. picture book of herself and the styles she has worn over the years
    C. employment portfolio showing before and after photos of past clients
    D. picture book of the type of salon and layout she prefers to work in

26. In order to validate her claim that she has been a responsible employee while working for others, Amira should provide:
    A. letters of commendation from her school
    B. a trophy she won in high school
    C. letters of reference from past employers
    D. old pay stubs

27. After having met and spent some time with the salon manager, Amira should send:
    A. a bouquet of flowers
    B. a state board inspector into the salon
    C. a basket of muffins
    D. a "thank-you" note for the interview

28. If she is offered the position, Amira will have to decide _____ before taking the job.
    A. if the salon has enough shampoo bowls to accommodate all of the salon's needs
    B. if the stylists she'll be working with are candidates for possible friendship
    C. if the salon has the kind of image, culture, and values that she has
    D. if the color palette the designer used to decorate the salon is suitable to her tastes

Chapter 26

ON THE JOB

OUT IN THE REAL WORLD

Today is Marshall's first day at the Jolie Salon and he is excited. He will meet the entire staff this morning at the weekly staff meeting, and then he'll meet with Sara, the salon manager, to go over the rules and regulations of the salon and of his financial remuneration. Marshall also has a few questions he wants to ask Sara and a couple of issues he would like her to clarify.

29. Sara tells Marshall that the salon operates very much like a/an ____ in that everyone is aware of his own duties but is also ready and must be willing to aid coworkers in whatever needs to be accomplished.
    A. booth rental situation
    B. team
    C. individual salon
    D. private salon

30. Sara explains that payday is on Friday and that he will make a ____, which is a percentage of his service dollars and an hourly wage.
    A. commission
    B. salary
    C. tip
    D. salary plus commission

31. Sara explains that after his first 90 days of employment, Marshall will have a/an ____, which will be an opportunity for her to assess his progress and performance and for Marshall to discuss his thoughts and ideas about the salon.
    A. hair service
    B. employee evaluation
    C. in-salon training class
    D. management workshop

32. Marshall asks Sara if she can help him determine what his paychecks might be for the first three months of employment so that he can make a ____ to track his expenses such as loan repayments and household expenses.
    A. salon budget
    B. pie chart of client retention
    C. personal budget
    D. tipping sheet

33. Sara assigns Marshall to Joyce, a senior stylist, who will be responsible for answering his questions, giving him guidance, and helping him when he has difficulty. Joyce will be his:
    A. friend
    B. coworker
    C. manager
    D. mentor

Sheniqwa has just learned that her salon will be retailing a product line that she has used in the past and has wanted to sell to her clients for some time. She is excited because many of the salon's clients can really benefit from the products and the new services their use will introduce to the salon. Sheniqwa's first client is Noreen who has had her hair colored and chemically straightened, and who uses a hot iron to flatten and style her hair about once a week. As a result of the intense chemicals and heat, Noreen's hair is very brittle, dry and damaged, and Sheniqwa feels that any additional pulling or styling may cause Noreen's hair to break.

34. When Noreen comes in for her haircut and styling appointment, Sheniqwa should:
    A. get reacquainted with Noreen and proceed with the service
    B. offer Noreen a cup of coffee and walk her to the styling station
    C. fill Noreen in on all of the latest gossip since her last visit
    D. review Noreen's record card and discuss the condition of her hair

35. While discussing her hair, Noreen mentions that she is having difficulty with her hair being so dry and looking so dull. Sheniqwa will want to use this as an opportunity to:
    A. discuss the new line of retail products to Noreen and how they can benefit her
    B. tell her what a mistake it is to chemically straighten the hair
    C. talk her into leaving her hair curly and natural
    D. suggest that she wear a wig for a while

36. Since Noreen's hair is very dry and damaged, Sheniqwa suggests adding a deep conditioning treatment to today's service. This is called:
    A. upping the service
    B. ticket upgrading
    C. adding up the ticket
    D. selling unneeded services

37. Once Noreen has had her service and sees the benefit of the treatment, Sheniqwa can use a _____ approach to recommending additional retail products for at-home use.
    A. hard sell
    B. fast sell
    C. soft sell
    D. slow sell

Cassie is worried. She has a great clientele who are very loyal to her, but she knows that if she moves to a bigger salon and rents more space, her expenses will go up and she wonders what she can do to increase her income. She decides to take some time and write out her plan for how to increase her income to cover her expenses by increasing her client base. Cassie gets to work.

38. In order to obtain important demographic information on her clients, Cassie will need to refer to her:
    A. salon manual
    B. client record cards
    C. appointment book
    D. technical literature

39. Cassie notes that she can use her business cards to:
    A. get speaking engagements
    B. promote a referral program with current clients
    C. obtain free entrance to hair shows
    D. impress new clients with her professionalism

40. As a reward for her loyal clients, and to promote the purchase of additional services and products, Cassie can prepare a ____ and include it in a "thank you" or birthday card mailing.
    A. free bottle of nail polish
    B. CD of the music played in the salon
    C. discount coupon
    D. gift certificate for a lunch at a nearby restaurant

41. To make herself visible to new groups of potential clients, Cassie could:
    A. work harder at keeping her current client base
    B. steal clients from other stylists in her current salon
    C. make herself available to speak at local organizations
    D. stake out neighboring salons and hand out flyers to their clients

42. Cassie could make use of her relationships with other local merchants by:
    A. going to their place of business and secretly handing out her business card
    B. agreeing to cross-promote with merchants who are willing to do so
    C. working part time in their establishment
    D. discouraging her clients from using local merchants

43. Cassie realizes that one of the simplest ways to increase her business is to:
    A. double her prices
    B. listen to clues clients give and offer services to accommodate their needs
    C. use a less expense brand of shampoo and conditioner
    D. purchase haircolor and perm solution in bulk

ANSWER KEY

Part I—Orientation

Chapter 2

LIFE SKILLS

THE PSYCHOLOGY OF SUCCESS

1. John's self-esteem appears to be based on:
   B. *His ability to possess things*
      True self-esteem is based on inner strength and trusting your ability to reach your goals. Since John's is based on his ability to possess things, his self-esteem will be dictated by how many things or belongings he has. This is not a real assessment of who John is or what his value and worth are.

2. John has used the technique of visualization to:
   A. *Picture himself as a complete success*
      Visualization is a technique John can use to see himself in a certain light in his mind's eye, which makes it easier for him to manifest the image into reality because he is adept at seeing it, feeling it, and being comfortable with it.

3. A truly successful person does not:
   C. *Allow business to be the only focus of his life*
      A truly successful person works hard but also takes time to enjoy the fruits of his labor such as friendship, family, rest and relaxation, and quiet time to reflect and think about his life.

4. John's lifestyle requires him to spend all of his time:
   D. *Working*
   > John has created a very rigid lifestyle that does not allow him to do any of the things he may really enjoy such as visiting with family and friends, exercising, or exploring hobbies.

5. John's definition of success includes:
   D. *Keeping up appearances*
   > A balanced view of success includes not only financial success but also the ability to have time for both work and pleasure, continuing to learn, and having time daily for exercise and caring for the physical as well as emotional body.

6. Whose definition of success is John attempting to achieve?
   C. *His client's*
   > John feels that in order to be respected and patronized by this elite clientele, he must be seen by them as one of them. He thinks his equality is based on the possession and acquisition of material things.

TIME MANAGEMENT

7. The first thing Ramona must do is:
   B. *Prioritize the list of tasks that need to be done in the order of most to least important*
   > With a priority list of tasks that need to be accomplished, Ramona can be sure that the most important ones are being attended to and that they are not superceded by less important tasks.

8. Ramona needs to have some specific time with her young child each day. She can accomplish this by:
   B. *Designing a schedule for herself that includes blocks of unstructured time*
   > If Ramona created a time management structure she followed daily, she could be sure that those things that are of the greatest importance receive the kind of

time they need and deserve. This way, important tasks and appointments aren't shortchanged.

9. Which of the following will NOT save Ramona time in her busy schedule?

    C. *Relying on others to problem-solve and uncover solutions she can use*

    Ramona will waste a lot of time if she needs to check and double check decisions with others before she acts. By using a priority list and a time management system, Ramona can be well aware of her needs and the options available to her so that she can act quickly and expediently.

10. When Ramona is feeling overwhelmed by the circumstances of her hectic life, she could try a technique called:

    B. *Deep breathing*

    By taking a moment or two to calm herself down, Ramona can concentrate on the demands at the moment and open herself to the many possibilities for a solution to her dilemma. Deep breathing or meditating is one way to stop the mind from wandering and to get focused.

11. To aid Ramona in remembering important notes and reminders, she should carry:

    A. *A memo pad or day planner*

    Many people find it very helpful to have a dedicated place to jot down notes and reminders as they think of them, and to always keep their notes in the same place,. A memo pad or day planner also cuts down on the incidence of losing an important note or reminder.

12. Ramona might consider scheduling her time in ____ intervals to study for a major exam.

    D. *60-minute*

    By scheduling one hour increments of time for studying, Ramona allows herself enough time to settle into studying, to make notes, and review material without interruption or without spending so much time that she becomes bored or anxious.

13. To make the most of her time, Ramona should schedule activities that require alert, clear thinking during times when she is:

   C. *Highly energetic and able to focus*

   Trying to accomplish tasks at the end of the day when she is tired, or after a great amount of physical or mental energy has been expended on something else, is a time-waster. Ramona should know what type of energy level is needed for her various tasks and schedule them at those times during the day when it is most conducive to the task.

14. Which of the following is NOT a healthy way for Ramona to reward herself for a job well done?

   D. *Smoking a cigarette*

   Ramona should reward herself for doing a good job but the method she uses should be one that enhances her mental, physical, and spiritual self instead of doing something that is potentially harmful or dangerous to herself and her well-being.

15. Another activity Ramona must consider scheduling to promote clear thinking and planning is:

   A. *Exercising*

   By planning some physical exercise everyday— walking, running, or going to a gym—Ramona is taking good care of her physical well-being and doing what she can to maintain a good, healthy, and strong body.

16. Which of the following tools would help Ramona the most to keep herself focused on the tasks she needs to complete each day?

   C. *A to-do list*

   A to-do list will help Ramona stay on track and abreast of the tasks that need to be accomplished each day. A to-do list is especially useful for her to carry around with her and to check throughout the day when she has additional time to knock off one or two tasks.

STUDY SKILLS

17. What is missing from Hector's educational background?
    B. *Good study skills*
       Hector didn't have the opportunity to learn some of the basics of how to study such as staying focused on the task at hand and resisting distractions during those times that he has set aside for study. These are tools he can learn to make studying easier for himself.

18. When Hector feels overwhelmed by his courses and upcoming tests, he can focus on ____ to feel better about himself and his progress.
    C. *Accomplishing small tasks, one at a time*
       Trying to do something new, and becoming proficient and successful at it, can be very difficult and frustrating. Hector should break down each task into several smaller tasks and focus on accomplishing them one at a time. Sooner than later he will have the entire goal accomplished and realize that he is able to do whatever he sets his mind to doing.

19. Instead of cramming the night before an exam, Hector should:
    D. *Study the day's lessons each day, then review all the material before the exam*
       By using a time management system while he is in school, and by scheduling an hour or so each day to review the day's lessons and readings, Hector will slowly build up his knowledge of material he is studying as well as his self-confidence as a student and learner.

20. Which of the following techniques will help Hector stay focused when his mind begins to wander in class?
    C. *Write down key words and discuss them with the instructor*
       In a classroom where there are many people and many activities are happening simultaneously, it is

easy to become distracted and to lose focus on the lesson at hand. Hector can make notes of things he wants to discuss further, words or phrases he didn't understand, or techniques he would like to see demonstrated again, and use these notes to check in with his instructor. By letting these missed opportunities slip by without further discussion, Hector risks missing chunks of information or concepts that other material will build on.

21. If Hector decides to form and/or join a study group, what should he look for in the group?
   B. *Students who are willing to be helpful and supportive*
      Too many people join study groups because they want to enjoy the company, friendship, or camaraderie of a group of peers. While friendship can certainly be a pleasant side effect of a study group, one should choose a group that has the resources to provide an environment for learning and enhancing the learning experience.

22. If Hector was to find a "study buddy," what would that person's job be?
   C. *To help him stay focused on studying*
      A study buddy is someone who would work with Hector and help him focus on the lessons of the day, week, and semester. This person should be someone that Hector could discuss ideas and concepts with, and someone who would make it a priority to work with Hector to aid him in concentrating on his studies.

LEARNING STYLES

23. What type of learner is Janice?
   B. *Reader/listener learner*
      Reader/listener learners learn best by reading and hearing new ideas, then mulling them over in their minds. They have a great memory for facts and details and they are eager to know the reasons for things.

24. What type of learner is Delores?
    D. *Intuitive learner*
       Intuitive learners like to get their hands into the learning process, and they learn best by trying it out and doing it.

25. What type of learner is James?
    A. *Interactive learner*
       Interactive learners learn best when they can participate in the process, and they like to discuss the situation with other students and instructors.

26. What type of learner is Jill?
    C. *Systematic learner*
       Systematic learners love to know how things will work and they want to have real-life situations that depict the lesson they are learning.

27. A reader/listener learner is someone who asks the question:
    B. *What*
       Since these learners are eager to know the reasons for things, they often ask themselves and their teachers "What will happen if . . . ?"

28. Intuitive learners like to learn through:
    A. *Trial and error*
       Intuitive learners want to do it themselves so they will often not truly understand a concept until they can try to accomplish the task and assess the outcome.

29. Interactive learners most appreciate instructors who are:
    C. *Sympathetic and friendly*
       Since these learners want to be involved in the learning experience, their instructors must make a special effort to allow them to be active in and carried away by the process.

30. Systematic learners study best:
    C. *By themselves*
       Systematic learners study best by themselves because it is easier for them to concentrate on their own and to read and digest information.

ETHICS

31. In making his decision, Adam must choose the person who is best at:

    C. *Honestly speaking to stylists*
       Keeping a salon staff happy and keeping a salon running smoothly requires the skills of a person who is open and able to communicate and relate to others honestly. A good manager, while not perfect, does his best to balance all of the responsibilities.

32. In assessing Hakim and Jake, which of the following does NOT indicate a high standard of professionalism?

    B. *Avoiding all conflict*
       While dealing with conflict is the least pleasant thing a manager has to do, it is among the most important things. All too often, in an effort to avoid the unpleasantness of conflict, people simply do not address situations and resolve them in a timely manner, which only creates an opportunity for bigger problems the longer they remain unresolved.

33. Which of the following is NOT an ethical characteristic for Hakim and Jake to aspire to?

    D. *Uncooperativeness*
       There are times in every person's career when they feel they have to take a stand and even perhaps disagree with the way a decision is being made, but consciously deciding to be uncooperative is nothing more than an immature approach to handling conflict and amounts to sabotaging the group's effectiveness.

34. Based on Jake's behavior, what type of personality traits is he likely displaying when he is asked to manage the salon?

    B. *A difficult, disagreeable personality*
       When Jake is asked to manage the salon, his behavior indicates that he is immature and a bit power hungry. He becomes bossy and rude to his fellow stylists, which fosters an environment of chaos instead of cohesion, and this is dangerous in large doses.

35. As a caregiver, Hakim must be able to practice:
    B. *Self-care*
        Hakim, like any caregiver—doctors, nurses, therapists—will only be able to give excellent care if he feels perfectly taken care of himself. This means that he must be sure to tend to his physical, psychological, and emotional needs, and to know himself and his limits well enough to know when he needs to be recharged.

36. When determining Jake and Hakim's sense of integrity, Adam will need to assess:
    B. *If their behavior and actions match their values*
        Many people can use catch words and popular phrases, or can say what they think another person will want to hear, but the true test of a person's integrity is when you observe his behavior and actions, the things that indicate what the person really values.

37. For Jake to display a good sense of integrity, he would have to behave in the following manner:
    D. *Recommend products and services from which the client can benefit*
        While selling in and of itself isn't a bad thing, professionals have to remember that they have trained and worked hard to achieve their position as trusted resources for their clients, and to betray that trust in any way is to trade in their long-term success and happiness for a short-lived commission.

38. When Jake gossips with other stylists about a client's personal situation, he is lacking:
    C. *Discretion*
        When Jake became a cosmetologist, he became a person that his colleagues and clients alike began to confide in. People told him private and confidential information about themselves and their preferences. Along with the information he received, he made an unspoken promise not to use the information in any way that could be hurtful and damaging to the person

who confided in him. When Jake gossips about himself or others, he lacks good judgment.

39. Which of the following characteristics indicates that Hakim is extending ethical behavior to his communication with customers and the other people with whom he works?

    C. *Being direct*

    So much miscommunication can occur when people do not say what they actually mean. Being direct with the people that you are in communication with can go a long way toward having an experience that is honest and focused. Being coy or indirect usually confuses the situation and causes hard feelings.

PERSONALITY DEVELOPMENT AND ATTITUDE

40. From her response, what kind of attitude does Marcia have about people who are late?

    C. *She is impatient and distrusting*

    One of Marcia's most important jobs is to keep the flow of the salon moving; however, hectic lives inevitably mean that clients will need to change appointments. While she may be annoyed that Mr. Hatch inconvenienced her and the stylist, she must also remember that their salon can only be successful if they accommodate their clients' needs.

41. How would you rate Marcia's ability to handle the situation with Mr. Hatch tactfully?

    C. *Fair—she wasn't very sympathetic but managed to reschedule the client*

    While she was able to reschedule the appointment, she did not present the salon in a very friendly or sympathetic manner to the client. While he will likely keep his appointment, the burden now falls more heavily on the stylist to repair anything that may have been lost in the delicate relationship between the client and the salon.

42. How should Marcia have handled the conversation with Mr. Hatch?

   D. *She should have let him know that missing his appointment was a problem, and asked him if he'd prefer to be the last client of the day to give him ample time to get to the salon*

   A useful technique for clients who are chronically late or for those who have to drive a long distance in traffic is to give them the last appointment of the day so that if they are late or if they have to cancel altogether, the effect on the stylist's schedule is minimized.

43. How sensitive was Marcia to Mr. Hatch?

   D. *Not sensitive at all*

   Marcia's attitude and responses to Mr. Hatch conveyed that she was more concerned about her own inconvenience and that of the stylist than to the needs of the client.

44. Based on Marcia's response to this situation, what do you think her values and goals are?

   D. *Accusation and blame*

   Since Marcia is in a position that can be stressful, and since every missed or mishandled appointment has a financial impact on the salon, it is easy to see how Marcia may want the stylist and her salon manager to know that she was not to blame for the incident with Mr. Hatch. However, becoming accusatory and/or blaming will only serve to alienate a good client from the salon.

45. What will likely be the effect of Marcia's comments on Mr. Hatch?

   D. *He will feel guilty*

   While it is likely that Mr. Hatch will keep his appointment, it is almost a certainty that he will feel embarrassed, reprimanded, and even angry because a simple situation was made much larger than it had to be. Even if the client agrees to continue to come to the salon, there is likely to be a negative residue overshadowing the experience for quite some time to come.

HUMAN RELATIONS

46. Tyrone's reaction to Eva indicated that he was:
    C. *Unprepared for her complaints and took them personally*
        Since Eva was not the first client to lodge this complaint, and since he apparently already looked into the problem at his company, Tyrone has no excuse for not being prepared for this. He took her impatience as a personal insult when she was simply frustrated and disappointed in the customer service she was receiving.

47. If Tyrone had a strong sense of his abilities, how would he have behaved with Eva?
    D. *He would call her with a delivery date and propose some alternative options*
        Since Tyrone had plenty of time to either get a date for when the items would be delivered or to have come up with a backup plan to accommodate his client, he should have been better able to handle her needs. If he was unsure about how best to serve the client, Tyrone could have checked in with his sales manager for advice and more options to offer Eva.

48. Had Tyrone really been listening to Eva's complaint, what opportunity might he have been presented with?
    A. *The chance to sell her a new product line to try*
        An adept salesperson is someone who is always ready to offer solutions to his customer's problems. In this scenario, Tyrone became part of the problem instead of part of the solution, and in doing so, he missed an opportunity to help the client and to make an additional sale.

49. What would have been the best way for Tyrone to attend to Eva's needs?
    C. *Agree with her complaint and ask what he could do to help her in the short term*

    Eva needed to vent her frustrations, so as her sales consultant, it was appropriate for him to allow her to complain a bit. Once she was allowed to do some of that, Tyrone is trained to redirect the conversation into more constructive and useful directions.

50. From Tyrone's reaction to Eva, what can you infer about his job satisfaction?
    D. *He is unhappy at work and is not handling his frustrations in a positive manner*

    If Tyrone is unhappy, frustrated, or angry about the circumstances under which he works, he needs to find a mature way of handling his feelings and resolving his problems before he can really be of service to his own customers.

Chapter 3

YOUR PROFESSIONAL IMAGE

BEAUTY AND WELLNESS

51. Does it sound like Marcella is enjoying good health?
    D. *No, her mind, body, and spirit do not seem to be working cooperatively*
        Marcella seems to be overly stressed out and tired, and based on her schedule and her apparent living situation, she is just barely managing her affairs.

52. One of the most important things that Marcella seems to be lacking is:
    A. *Balance*
        Marcella is well aware that she needs to work but she has chosen to make her work the number one priority in her life, neglecting her personal appearance and health. Living a more balanced life would help Marcella give equal attention to her person as well as to her work situation.

53. Based on the reaction from Marcella's colleagues, how would you rate her personal hygiene?
    D. *Fair*
        We all know how unpleasant an experience it can be to be in contact with someone who has body odor or bad breath. If the condition is so bad that people are actually pulling away from her when in conversation, a simple solution is available to Marcella such as using freshening towelettes throughout the day.

54. Which of the following should Marcella NOT do to improve her personal hygiene between jobs?
    D. *Douse herself with perfume*
        Sometimes, when people are in a rush, they may opt to take what they consider the easiest solution. In

this case, dousing oneself with perfume or cologne will not really resolve the body odor issue but will probably make it more pronounced. Instead of covering up, all Marcella needs to do is freshen up.

55. What is most likely the cause of coworkers and clients pulling away from her when Marcella is speaking to them?

   C. *Bad breath*

   Most likely, Marcella has bad breath. If she is aware of her propensity for it, she can keep some toothpaste and a toothbrush in her handbag or tucked away in her station so that she can freshen up during the day when she needs to.

56. What does Marcella's disheveled appearance say about her professionalism?

   D. *That she is feeling stress and cannot manage her time*

   Marcella's appearance says that she is overwhelmed by her life and her working conditions, and she is not taking proper care of herself and her health, and, therefore, not acting in a manner befitting a professional person.

57. How should Paige go about finding the best place to work?

   A. *Visit several salons and determine which one is most in line with her own sense of style*

   While Paige probably needs a job very badly, the worst thing she can do is make herself into someone she is not to get a job. She should visit several salons in her area, those that most align with the kind of tastes and preferences she has, then decide which of those she would like to work in.

58. What is the energy and image of the spa Paige is interviewing at?

   C. *A high-end spa that has an exclusive clientele*

   A luxury spa is definitely an environment that caters to affluent clients who are willing to spend their money on luxury products and services, and who will expect to be serviced by a certain type of

professional whose personal style mirrors the spa's and their own.

59. What type of salon seems most appropriate for someone with Paige's sense of style to work in?

   B. *A moderately priced salon that caters to young clients who have a sense of adventure*

   To be successful in the long term, Paige needs to work in a salon whose style reflects her own and that caters to clients who can appreciate her sense of style.

60. Is Paige's approach to getting this job ethical?

   C. *No, because she isn't being honest about who she really is*

   A major component of being ethical is being honest in all of the aspects of each dealing. By dressing and acting like the other stylists in the salon, then intending to resume her preferred style after she gets the job, Paige is not being honest with the spa owners or with herself.

61. The best time for Allie to approach Peter would be:

   C. *When they are alone in the salon*

   Allie wants to discuss this very personal issue with Peter and so the best time to speak to him is when they are alone so that he is not embarrassed or distracted by others. In this way, she will have the best chance of being able to get through to Peter.

62. What should Allie discuss with Peter?

   A. *His personal appearance and its affect on the salon's clients*

   Allie must keep the conversation focused and professional and not allow her personal feelings or judgments to get interjected. Allie is responsible for the smooth operation of the salon, and it is perfectly acceptable for her to discuss his behavior and appearance with Peter.

63. What could Peter do to make sure he is fresh for work, even on nights when he doesn't sleep at home?

   C. *Keep clean clothing in his car and freshen up before arriving at the salon*

   No matter what else is happening in Peter's life, he should make his professional appearance and demeanor a priority. By keeping fresh clothing in his car or by awakening early enough to go home and get dressed in clean clothing, he can handle the issue directly.

64. The image that Peter is projecting to clients suggests that he is:
B. *Between apartments and sleeping wherever he can*
Peter is not portraying himself as a serious or dedicated professional; rather, he looks like someone who is sloppy and careless. No client will want to subject herself to someone like Peter more than once or twice. Not only will Peter lose clients, but so will the salon.

HEALTHY MIND AND BODY

65. Carol seems to have an abundance of _____ in her life.
C. *Stress*
Carol feels stress because she is in a position to manage several things, people, and situations she really has very little control over.

66. To alleviate her stress, Carol should consider:
C. *Making time to sit quietly each day and connecting with her spiritual self*
Making it a habit of sitting quietly for a few minutes a day or several times a day will help Carol to calm down, relax a bit throughout the day, and be better equipped to handle the day-to-day issues that will come up as she manages the salon and her family life.

67. When in the middle of a stressful situation, Carol should:
B. *Take a couple of deep breaths to get herself centered* .
Using a deep breathing technique can be very effective to create a pause between the action and the reaction. Those few seconds can give Carol enough time to calm herself down and think up a constructive solution.

68. How is Carol currently handling her stress?
    C. *She is becoming impatient and snapping at others*
         Carol is obviously frustrated by what is occurring in
         her life, and without allowing herself the time and the
         opportunity to process her feelings, her emotions are
         inappropriately directed at others.

69. In order to handle her stress, Carol may need to create
    more _____ in her life.
    A. *Balance*
         Carol definitely needs to find a way to work
         through her thoughts and feelings about all of the
         various situations in her life. Because her schedule is
         so hectic, she has probably not given herself the time
         to work through her emotions about the changes in
         her life circumstances.

70. In order to reduce her stress, Carol should try to:
    B. *Get more sleep*
         Anytime someone is under acute stress, he may
         have difficulty sleeping or relaxing, and a lack of rest
         will have a profound affect on that person's
         disposition. Carol probably not only needs to get
         more sleep but also to find other ways to relax her
         mind and body throughout the day.

71. Which of the following could Carol do on a daily basis to
    relax?
    C. *Take a walk*
         Taking a few minutes a day to get some moderate
         physical exercise can really help clear people's minds
         and give them a few minutes to refocus their energies
         and thoughts. Getting exercise can mean joining a
         gym or just deciding to walk instead of drive to
         complete errands.

72. If Johnnie wants to improve how he is feeling, what
    should he do?
    C. *Eat a nutritionally balanced diet*
         Everyone needs to be conscious of the food and
         nutrients they are putting into their bodies. Since
         cosmetology is a physically demanding profession,

beauty professionals must be especially careful to treat their bodies to good, nutritious food.

73. In order to lose the extra weight that he's gained, Johnnie needs to consider:
     B. *Adding some moderate exercise to his day*
         Many people want to lose weight quickly so they turn to "quick-fixes" that don't really work and certainly can't be sustained. To lose weight and keep it off, Johnnie needs to commit to moving his body every day or every other day.

74. In order to maintain a healthy weight, Johnnie will need to monitor:
     A. *Snacking on junk food*
         There is an old saying, "Everything in moderation," and it means that a little bit of something is okay, but whenever you overdo it on one thing, you run the risk of hurting yourself. This is certainly the case with high fat foods and snack foods. Johnnie may want to allow himself some of his favorites, but he will need to limit the amount he has and the frequency with which he has them.

75. When Johnnie is waiting for his potential clients to become available, which of the following could he be doing to relieve his frustrations and stress?
     A. *Meditating*
         If Johnnie is truly hungry, he should make it a priority to schedule a lunch break so that he can have a proper meal. But if he is eating out of boredom or stress, he can find it very pleasurable and relaxing to meditate while waiting. Meditating will help reenergize him and get him ready for his work.

76. What percentage of his daily caloric intake should Johnnie be receiving from fat calories?
     C. *30%*
         Consuming too much fat from fast food or snack foods can contribute to a number of weight-related

health problems, and generally make a person feel
terrible.

77. Which of the following would be a healthy choice for
Johnnie to choose for lunch?
  B. *A low-fat sandwich on a multigrain roll with fresh fruit*
      By eating this meal, Johnnie will be satisfied, and
      he will be eating a low-fat and nutritious lunch that
      will certainly sustain him for the bulk of the
      afternoon.

YOUR PHYSICAL PRESENTATION

78. What does Marilyn's physical presentation indicate?
  B. *Poor posture*
      Marilyn's posture, the way that she holds herself, is
      being compromised by her lack of attention to how
      she is contorting her body while at work. She
      probably wants to be comfortable during her work
      hours but doesn't realize that she is hurting herself by
      holding her body in this manner.

79. To achieve and maintain a good standing posture, in
what position should Marilyn's head and neck be?
  C. *Level with the floor*
      She should keep her head level with the floor to
      ensure that she doesn't strain her neck or back by
      leaning too far forward or backward.

80. To relieve the tension in her shoulders, Marilyn should:
  B. *Level and relax them*
      This technique not only relaxes the shoulders but
      also allows the muscles to be lightly stretched and
      then relaxed, causing the tension to dissipate.

81. When standing, in what position should Marilyn's spine
be?
  D. *Perfectly straight*
      To prevent unnecessary and painful damage to her
      back, Marilyn should try to keep her spine as straight
      as possible as she can throughout the day.

82. A sitting posture that would alleviate Marilyn's back and neck pain would include:
    C. *Keeping her back straight*

    Keeping her back straight even when sitting may be tricky as nail techs tend to become so involved in the service they are performing that they forget to be aware of their posture. But it will be the only real way to prevent back pain and damage.

83. If it is necessary for Marilyn to bend forward, which part of her body should be bent?
    D. *Hips*

    Bending at the hips will give Marilyn the exact position she needs to perform her service, while also allowing her to maintain a healthy posture and not put undue stress on her back, neck, and shoulders.

84. How can Marilyn make her work environment more ergonomically correct for herself?
    B. *She can adjust the client's chair*

    Adjusting the client's chair to suit the needs of the stylist or nail tech is exactly the reason that client chairs are adjustable. The client should be seated in the chair and an assessment of adjustments can be made. Then the client should stand up so the adjustments can be made, then seated again. Never make adjustments to a chair while the client is seated in the chair.

85. To relieve muscle fatigue from standing for long periods, Marilyn could try:
    A. *Standing on a cushioned mat*

    Standing on a softer surface while working will ease the tension she'll hold in her body and be a bit easier on her leg and back muscles.

Chapter 4

COMMUNICATING FOR SUCCESS

COMMUNICATION BASICS

86. When Victoria first walked into the salon, what had she neglected to do?

C. *Collect her thoughts*

Victoria entered the salon on impulse and hadn't really thought about what she would say or ask for. She hadn't gathered her thoughts and translated them into a question; rather, she felt an emotion—I hate my hair—and acted on the feeling without being ready to verbalize her needs.

87. When Victoria told Abe that she needed help with her hair, how did Abe help her articulate her thoughts more clearly?

D. *By asking her questions*

An effective communication tool is to ask questions, especially if the person with whom you are communicating needs more time to gather her thoughts. By asking her questions, Abe was able to help Victoria pinpoint her thoughts. Then they were able to have an open and useful conversation.

88. How did Victoria clarify her desires to Abe?

B. *By showing him a photo in a magazine*

Sometimes the old adage is correct: a picture is worth a thousand words. By using the photo in the magazine, Victoria was able to quickly and clearly articulate to Abe what she was trying to achieve, and the result was a concise understanding.

89. When Abe describes the attributes of the style she has selected back to Victoria, he is using a technique called:

C. *Reflective listening*

Using the reflective listening technique is a valuable tool for professional cosmetologists because it allows the two people in the communication exchange the opportunity to hear and get clarification on what is being said.

90. Based on the exchange between Abe and Victoria, what is the outcome likely to be?
    D. *Victoria may return to the salon and request Abe's services*
       Employing good communication skills is one of the best ways for a stylist to convey to a client that he is interested in her needs, and is willing and able to understand and accommodate her needs.

91. By going the extra mile to fully understand Victoria's needs, Abe was attempting to build a strong _____.
    A. *Relationship*
       The outcome of any good communications exchange is to either begin a new or strengthen an existing relationship. Successful cosmetology careers are built on strong relationships between clients and their stylists.

THE CLIENT CONSULTATION

92. Dennis plans to equip the consultation area with the following furniture:
    C. *Comfortable chairs and table*
       It is important to have a consultation area that is attractive and inviting, and to furnish it with furniture that is comfortable. Chairs that make sitting in them a positive experience and a table that allows the people in the consultation to have enough room to look at books and magazines is exactly what is necessary.

93. Which of the following materials is NOT necessary for Dennis to provide during a client consultation?
    A. *A telephone*
       The consultation area should not only be comfortable but should also be private and free from any type of disturbance, which includes a ringing

telephone. During the consultation, both the client and the stylist should turn their phones off, and should understand that taking calls interrupts the conversation and the experience.

94. What type of atmosphere should Dennis provide for the room to be most conducive while speaking to clients about their services?

C. *A quiet, well-lit room so clients can adequately participate in the conversation*

   The area must be quiet so that the participants can concentrate on the conversation and the room must be well-lit so that the participants can really see what colors they are agreeing to. Dennis has opted to use the client card (Figure 4–7) for all of his salon's client consultations. Use the card as a basis for answering the following questions.

95. Having clients fill in all of the questions pertaining to their address and other personal information allows Dennis' salon to:

B. *Correctly identify each client*

   Many people share the same last name, and since they may not be related or share the same household, having clients fill in all of the pertinent information is an easy way to differentiate among them.

96. Knowing when the client last visited a salon will help the stylists in Dennis' salon to:

B. *Assess the client's commitment to her style's upkeep*

   This is a crucial element to a client remaining satisfied with her look and ultimately, her choice of salon. Stylists can use the record card and the client's style history to make recommendations for streamlining or adding to a client's routine to make the experience a positive and pleasant one.

Client Consultation Card

Dear Client,

Our sincerest hope is to serve you with the best hair care services you've ever received! We not only want you to be happy with today's visit but we also want to build a long-lasting relationship with you—we want to be your hair care salon. In order for us to do so, we would like to learn more about you, your hair care needs, and your preferences. Please take a moment now to answer the questions below as completely and as accurately as possible.

Thank you, and we look forward to building a "beautiful" relationship!

Name: _____

Address: _____

Address: _____

Phone Number: _____ (day) _____ (evening) _____

Sex: _____ Male _____ Female _____ Age: _____

How did you hear about our salon?

If you were referred, who referred you?

Please answer the following questions in the space provided. Thanks!

1. Approximately when was your last salon visit?
2. In the past year, have you had any of the following services either in or out of a salon? (Please indicate the date on which you had it.)

   ____Haircut   ____ Full Head Lightening
   ____Haircolor   ____ Waxing (what type?)
   ____Permanent Wave or   ____ Manicure
        Texturizing Treatment   ____ Artificial Nail Services (please describe)
   ____Chemical Relaxing or   ____ Pedicure
        Straightening Treatment   ____ Facial/Skin Treatment
   ____Highlighting or Lowlighting   ____ Other (please list any other services you've
                                                       enjoyed at a salon that may not be listed
                                                       here).

3. Are you currently taking any medications? (Please list)
4. What is your natural hair color shade?
5. How would you describe your hair's texture?
6. How would you describe your hair's condition?
7. How would you describe the condition of your scalp?
8. What type of skin do you have? Dry _____ Oily _____ Normal _____ Combination _____
9. What type of skin care regimen do you follow? (Please explain) _____

   _____

10. How would you characterize your nails? Normal _____ Brittle _____ Flexible _____
11. Do you have any of the following nail services? (check all that apply) Silk wraps _____ Porcelain _____ Acrylic wraps _____ Glue manicure _____ Natural manicure _____ Paraffin hand treatments _____
12. Do you have any of the following foot services? (Check all that apply) Basic pedicure _____ Spa pedicure _____ Paraffin foot treatment _____
13. Do you ever experience dry, itchy skin? Scalp? If so, how often?
14. Do you notice that your ability to manage your hair, skin, or nail regimens change with the change in climate? How so?

(continued)

15. How often do you shampoo your hair?
16. How often do you condition your hair?
17. Once cleansed and conditioned, how do you style your hair?
18. Please list all of the products that you use on your hair, skin, and nails regularly.
19. On average, how much time do you spend each day styling your hair?
20. Are you now or have you ever been allergic to any of the products, treatments, or chemicals you've received during any salon service—hair, nails, or skin? (Please explain)
21. What is your biggest complaint concerning your hair?
22. What is your biggest complaint concerning your skin?
23. What is your biggest complaint concerning your nails?
24. What do you like about your hair?
25. What do you like about your complexion?
26. What do you like about your nails?
27. Please describe the best hairstyle you ever had and explain why you felt it was the best.
28. What is the one thing that you want your stylist to know about you/your beauty regimens?

NOTE: If this card was used in a beauty school setting, it would include a release form at the bottom such as the one below.

Statement of Release: I hereby understand that cosmetology students render these services for the sole purpose of practice and learning, and that by signing this form, I recognize and agree not to hold the school, its employees, or the student liable for my satisfaction or the service outcome.

Client Signature _____ Date _____

Service Notes

Today's Date:
Today's Services:
Notes:

Today's Date:
Today's Services:
Notes:

Today's Date:
Today's Services:
Notes:

Today's Date:
Today's Services:
Notes:

Today's Date:
Today's Services:
Notes:

Figure 4–7. Client Consultation Card

97. Asking clients which services they have had in the previous year allows the salon to:

D. *Determine the client's history and the hair's condition*

This is especially important for a client who is interested in having a chemical service on top of other chemical services she may have had previously. A stylist will want to know what other treatments a client has had so that he can best advise the client.

98. Why is it useful for Dennis to ask clients about the medications they take?

C. *So he can assess the effect of the medication on their beauty regime*

Many times, the medications a person takes won't have any affect on the beauty services being performed, but in some instances, certain treatments may need to be altered or watched carefully. A person with high blood pressure, for example, should not be left under the hairdryer for an extended period of time.

99. Dennis requires clients to answer questions about their skin and nail care because:

A. *He is opening a full-service salon*

It is best for a salon to get all of the pertinent information about clients the first time they come into the salon and fill in their client consultation cards. Since Dennis is opening a full-service salon, the likelihood that a client may have more than one type of service in the salon is great, so asking questions about the total beauty history is appropriate.

100. Why is it important for Dennis to know how often clients wash and condition their hair?

B. *So he can determine their hair care routine and suggest services that will work for them*

A stylist becomes a partner with her client in the care of her hair, and in so doing, earns the right to know about a client's habits and to recommend services and products that may be helpful and useful.

101. Asking clients about their allergies allows Dennis to:
   C. *Protect clients from products or services that may harm them*

   Knowing about a client's allergies is vital information in the fight to keep clients safe from ingredients that could seriously harm them.

102. Which of the following is exactly the type of information Dennis' stylists should include in the Service Notes section of the consultation card?
   D. *Any notes pertaining to the client's hair or its reaction during the service*

   It is crucial for a stylist to note any and all reactions a client's hair and skin may have during a service. This information not only protects the client from any harm but also may protect the salon from liability.

SPECIAL ISSUES IN COMMUNICATION

103. Based on this scenario, Angie's first impression of the salon is likely to be that it is:
   B. *Disorganized and too confused to make a new client feel comfortable*

   It is easy for a stylist who has been working in a salon for a long time to forget what it is like to be a newcomer, just as Marshall did here. He was so caught up in the day's activities that he overlooked the feelings of a new client, and he didn't take an important opportunity to welcome her to the salon and make her feel comfortable.

104. How should Marshall's assistant have greeted Angie?
   B. *With a smile and a handshake*

   Marshall's assistant was representing Marshall and the salon when she approached the new client, so she should have greeted her and made her feel welcomed and important.

105. When Angie arrived at the salon and checked in, what should the receptionist have offered to do?

C. *Give her a tour of the salon*

Even though she was busy, once she had handled whatever task she was working on at the reception desk when Angie walked in, the receptionist should have turned her attention to the new client. The receptionist should have greeted Angie, welcomed her, and then offered her a tour of the salon.

106. Although the salon was obviously busy, what could Marshall's assistant have done to help direct Angie?

B. *Wait for Angie to get up and accompany her to the shampoo area*

First, she should have been clued that this was a client new to the salon and that the receptionist had not had the opportunity to greet her properly or show her around. Then, with that insight, the assistant should have taken it upon herself to pick up the ball and properly initiate Angie to the salon, its layout and staff, and at the very least, wait for and accompany her to the shampoo area.

107. What should have been the first thing that Marshall said to Angie when he approached her?

A. *"Hi, my name is Marshall. Welcome to the salon."*

Marshall should have begun the conversation with Angie exactly the way he would begin any conversation: by introducing himself to her and by being genuinely happy to meet her.

HANDLING TARDY CLIENTS

108. Patti should handle the scheduling mixup by:

D. *Apologizing for the mixup and offering to reschedule the appointment*

Whether the client is correct or not, Patti's priority is to make the client feel important and to accommodate her needs. The best way to do this is to end the conversation about who is right and move on to when best to get the services scheduled.

109. If Kim insists that she needs her nail appointment today, what can Patti do to accommodate her request?
   B. *Check with Susan and reschedule Kim for an appointment at the end of the day*
       When a client has an urgent need, it is best to find a way to accommodate her as quickly as possible to avoid hard feelings. Even if the nail tech has a long day or has plans after her shift is scheduled to end, knowing that a client needs her may be enough incentive to make some changes that accommodate the client and end the problem.

110. In regard to Kim's remaining appointments, the salon should:
   A. *Be able to accommodate her eyebrow waxing and haircut appointments as scheduled*
       Kim's other appointments should be honored exactly as they were scheduled, and if possible, may present an opportunity to switch times to accommodate the manicure appointment that was missed.

111. If Kim is upset about not being able to have her nail service immediately, Patti should refer her to:
   D. *The salon's late policy*
       It is always better for the client-salon relationship to handle a scheduling mixup as quickly as possible, but if there continues to be an issue with the appointment, Patti can mention the salon's policy about missed appointments and then, again, offer to resolve the issue as soon as is feasible.

112. What could the salon easily do to confirm appointments for clients the evening before their appointments?
   B. *Call clients and confirm appointments*
       It is an excellent policy to call clients the evening before their appointments to remind them of the type of service they have booked and the time for which the appointment is scheduled. This also reminds clients to call the salon in case they have to cancel or reschedule the appointment.

113. Where is the best place for Ruth to have the conversation with Mrs. Mendez about what is wrong?
    D. *In the consultation area*
        Finding a private place to discuss the issues surrounding Mrs. Mendez's concerns is the best way to calm the client down and to have a moment for the stylist to regroup. The consultation area is also a private area and conducive to having an emotionally-charged conversation out of earshot of the other clients in the salon.

114. Which of the following most closely resembles a question that Ruth should be asking Mrs. Mendez?
    C. *"What specifically don't you like about the style?"*
        Ruth needs to get clarification from Mrs. Mendez about her thoughts and feelings about the style, and the best way to do this is by asking her client specific questions.

115. If Ruth is able to determine from Mrs. Mendez that she would prefer more layers cut into the style, what should Ruth do?
    D. *Schedule Mrs. Mendez for the next available appointment and recut her hair*
        At the earliest possible opportunity, Ruth should make the time to recut Mrs. Mendez's hair, and use that time to mend the miscommunication and attempt to salvage the client-stylist relationship.

116. In the areas around the head where it is already too short and more layers can't be cut into the style, Ruth must:
    C. *Honestly tell the client that they cannot be reshaped*
        It is very important for Ruth to be as polite and as sympathetic to Mrs. Mendez as she can be, but she must also be completely honest with her about every aspect of the haircut. If Ruth has any chance of mending her relationship with this client, she will need to be as open and up front as she can be.

117. If Ruth is not able to determine the source of Mrs. Mendez's dissatisfaction and they are not able to come to an amiable resolution, Ruth should:

A. *Call on her manager or a senior stylist for help and advice*

Sometimes, when there is a dispute between a client and a stylist, it is best to get an objective person to help and advise both parties. If Ruth is unable to please Mrs. Mendez, then calling on her manager or a senior stylist may be just what it takes to calm the client, and allow Ruth to satisfy Mrs. Mendez and rebuild the relationship.

118. How can Ruth use this experience to grow as a professional stylist?

A. *She can use the feedback to improve her service for the next client*

Although difficult and even unpleasant, Ruth should discuss this situation with her salon manager and/or mentor and ask them for honest and constructive feedback. Every stylist has encountered a similar situation in his career and can very likely offer Ruth good advice.

IN-SALON COMMUNICATION

119. Myrna's best course of action is to:

B. *Treat both stylists respectfully and fairly*

While there may be lots of reasons why certain stylists do or do not get along, Myrna needs to stay out of the argument and remain neutral. By showing each of the stylists respect and by treating them fairly without judgment, Myrna makes a statement about her integrity.

120. When asked whose side Myrna believes, she should:

D. *Remain neutral*

Myrna's best answer would have to be something like, "Since I wasn't involved in the situation, I really have no opinion one way or the other." This makes the statement that she is serious about remaining neutral.

121. If pushed into the conflict, what should Myna say to Bonnie and Stacy?

    D. *"I like you both and don't want to be involved in your argument"*

        If she is really pushed into it, Myrna must take a clear and concise stand on where she is with her feelings about getting into the middle of someone else's argument. She need not judge either of the stylists, and answering their question in this manner states that simply yet effectively.

122. If Myrna continues to feel pressured about taking a side, her best course of action is to ask ____ for help in resolving the matter.

    B. *Her salon manager*

        Anything that happens in the salon, especially something such as an argument where people are pressured into taking sides, is the responsibility of the salon manager. If Myrna cannot resolve this issue on her own, she always has a resource in her salon manager.

123. If Myna is feeling victimized about the pressure to get involved in the salon conflict, she may feel tempted to discuss it with other salon staff which would be:

    B. *Detrimental to maintaining a professional relationship at work*

        Gossiping or discussing private details of any situation at work is a bad idea, even in a case such as this one. If Myrna is feeling that she needs someone to talk with, she should choose to confide in someone other than a salon staffer—such as a friend or mentor—to get some of her frustrations out so that her feelings don't have an impact on her work life.

COMMUNICATING DURING AN EMPLOYEE EVALUATION

124. In preparation for the evaluation meeting, Bruce should think about and list:
     C. *Problems and possible solutions*
        Bruce will want to be open with his salon manager when he has his performance evaluation, but he must remember that she cannot solve every problem. Bruce should think about possible solutions to the problems he sees. This approach shows Bruce to be a proactive and motivated employee.

125. When discussing the issue of the construction outside of the salon and its effect on the salon's walk-in business, Bruce should:
     D. *Suggest some ideas for how to work around the inconvenience of the construction*
        The issue of the construction is likely to be a problem for the entire salon. If Bruce can suggest some possible solutions for working around it, he proves that he is a thinker, a leader, and someone who is worth looking to when an opportunity for management opens up.

126. When discussing the flex time policy and the fact that he is often left at the salon alone in the evening, Bruce needs to:
     D. *Ask for an explanation of the policy and how it should affect the evening shift*
        While Bruce may feel taken advantage of by other stylists who may abuse the flex time policy, it would be detrimental to his relationship with his manager, coworkers, and to his opportunity for promotion to simply go into his meeting and tattle on the other stylists. Instead, he should get clarification on the policy and then, if he is working with someone who he feels is abusing the policy, speak with them about it directly first before involving the salon manager.

127. When discussing any opportunities there may be for promotion, Bruce will need to be prepared to hear:

 B. *The areas that he will need to improve in order to be considered for a promotion*

 Anyone who is interested in becoming a manager must also be willing to improve his own skills, and be able to demonstrate that willingness to himself and the salon staff. Since, as a manager, he may be responsible for giving other employees feedback, Bruce will only be able to do this compassionately if he also learns how to give and receive feedback in order to be a good example to his coworkers.

128. If Bruce is serious about working toward a promotion, he will want to ask Jackie:

 A. *When they can meet again to discuss his progress*

 If it's really important to Bruce, he will be motivated to follow up with his manager and to work on improving those areas she outlines for him. While she may be willing to work with and train him for management, his progress will not be her most important priority, so Bruce will need to do his own follow-up.

129. Once the evaluation is completed, Bruce should ____ Jackie.

 A. *Thank*

 Preparing an employee evaluation and fairly delivering that evaluation is as much, if not more, work than being evaluated, so it would be polite for Bruce to express his gratitude to Jackie for her time and help.

Part II   Cosmetology Sciences

Chapter 5

INFECTION CONTROL: PRINCIPLES AND PRACTICE

BACTERIA

1. Mark appears to be spreading bacteria called:
   B. *Streptococci*
   > Streptococci are pus-forming bacteria that can cause strep throat and blood poisoning.

2. How might Cathy have been exposed to the bacteria that caused strep throat?
   B. *By breathing the same air as Mark*
   > Streptococci rarely are able to move about on their own; rather, they are transmitted in the air, in the dust, or within any substance in which they settle. By being in a confined space, Cathy could easily have contracted the bacteria from Mark by breathing the air he breathed.

3. Bacteria that is disease-causing is called:
   A. *Pathogenic*
   > A pathogenic bacterium is a harmful bacterium that can cause disease when it invades plant or animal tissue.

4. Strep throat is:
   D. *An infection*
   > An infection occurs when body tissues are invaded by disease-causing bacteria such as streptococci.

5. When Cathy looks inside of her mouth, she can see ____,
    which indicates that she has an infection.
    C. *Pus*
        Pus is a fluid product of inflammation, white blood
        cells, and the debris from dead cells, tissue elements,
        and bacteria. Its presence indicates infection.

6. Mark should:
    B. *Stay home from work to prevent the spread of disease*
        Since Mark is spreading disease, and since he has
        the opportunity to come into contact with many
        people each day, he should remain home in an effort
        to protect others from contracting the disease he is
        carrying.

7. A disease that can spread from Maureen to Mark to Cathy
    is said to be:
    B. *Communicable*
        A contagious disease, one that can be passed from
        person to person, is considered to be communicable.
        As cosmetologists, Mark and Cathy must be very
        aware that they could potentially expose clients and
        coworkers, and that they must take action to protect
        the public from the disease.

VIRUSES

8. What type of virus does Marlene likely have?
    B. *Hepatitis A*
        Hepatitis A usually lasts about three weeks. The
        symptoms mirror the flu and may cause a yellowing
        of the skin and eyes.

9. What type of virus does Sophia likely have?
    D. *Hepatitis C*
        Hepatitis C can progress slowly and infected
        persons may not always experience any symptoms.
        The most common symptoms include stomach pain
        and fatigue.

10. How is Marlene's virus usually spread?
    A. *By sharing an unsanitary restroom*
       Hepatitis A is spread through close household contact, poor sanitation, poor personal grooming, or infected food handlers.

11. How is Sophia's virus usually spread?
    A. *By having sexual relations with an infected person*
       This disease is spread by parenteral contact and sexual relations with infected partners. No vaccine is available for the treatment of Hepatitis C.

12. What organ is primarily affected by hepatitis?
    C. *The liver*
       Hepatitis is a disease marked by a inflammation of the liver and caused by a bloodborne pathogen virus that is present in all bodily fluids.

13. Which of the diseases listed below can be treated with a vaccine?
    B. *Hepatitis A*
       There is a vaccine available to combat Hepatitis A.

14. The disease-causing bacteria that are carried through Sophia's body are called:
    C. *Bloodborne pathogens*
       Bloodborne pathogens are disease-causing bacteria or viruses that are carried through the body by the blood or body fluids.

15. In order to protect others from the diseases they carry, both Marlene and Sophia should:
    B. *Immediately disinfect any implements that come in contact with their body fluids*
       Since both of these disease require a person to come into contact with body fluids to become infected, there is no need for Marlene or Sophia to stop working. However, they should be careful not to spread the bacteria by allowing other people to come into contact with their bodily fluids.

PARASITES

16. What is the yellow-green spot that Thomas has detected
    likely to be?
    C. *Fungi*
        Fungi are vegetable parasites that include mold,
        mildew, and yeasts, and can produce diseases such as
        ringworm and favus, both skin diseases.

17. Why can't Thomas remove the yellow-green spots he sees?
    A. *Because they are a skin disease*
        A skin disease is not a topical disease and, therefore,
        cannot simply be wiped away.

18. How could the fungus have been brought into the salon?
    B. *Gina may have had moisture trapped under a nail*
        A very common source of nail fungus is moisture
        that may become trapped or caught under a nail
        enhancement.

19. How could the fungus have spread from one client to
    another?
    A. *Improper disinfection of manicure implements*
        If an implement comes into contact with the fungus
        and then is not cleansed properly before being used on
        someone else, it may cause the spread of the fungus.

20. What is the most common treatment for a nail fungus?
    B. *Topical medication*
        In most cases, topical treatment is usually applied
        directly to the infected area, but in severe cases, a
        physician's care is required.

IMMUNITY

21. Both Lucille and Frank are attempting to enhance their
    ability to be ____ to/from disease.
    A. *Immune*
        Immunity is the ability of the body to ward off
        disease that has gained entrance to the body.

22. Frank's flu shot is considered to be:
   D. *An acquired immunity*
     An acquired immunity is an immunity the body develops after it overcomes a disease or after a vaccination.

23. Lucille's ability to stave off the flu by taking excellent care of herself is an example of someone with:
   A. *A natural immunity*
     Someone with a natural immunity has partly developed immunity through hygienic living but who also probably inherited it.

24. Which of the following can be credited with promoting natural immunity?
   B. *Washing hands frequently*
     Since our hands touch many things throughout the day—things that may or may not be infected with disease—washing our hands frequently keeps us from coming into contact with many types of disease. Hand-washing removes microorganisms from the folds and grooves of the skin by lifting and rinsing them from the skin's surface.

PRINCIPLES OF PREVENTION

25. In order to remove the pathogens and other substances that linger on the surfaces of the salon and on implements, the salon must be willing to:
   A. *Decontaminate*
     Decontamination is the removal of pathogens and other substances from surfaces and tools.

26. When Ginger's crew disinfects the salon, they are using chemical agents to destroy bacteria and viruses on:
   B. *Cutting implements*
     Disinfectants are used only on tools and surfaces and never on human skin because their strong chemicals can damage skin.

27. Ginger's crew follow MSDS and OSHA guidelines, which tell them:
    C. *How to properly store and dispose of the product*
    > Since these chemicals are dangerous to skin and could be dangerous if used improperly, it is imperative that anyone working with them handle them properly.

28. When Ginger considers the types of products for the crew to use, she must first decide if the product has the correct ____ for getting the job accomplished.
    C. *Efficacy*
    > A product's efficacy refers to its effectiveness at achieving the required results.

29. The cleaning crew may use a quat because it is:
    D. *Effective for cleaning countertops*
    > Quats, short for quaternary ammonium compounds, are types of disinfectants considered nontoxic, odorless, and fast-acting, and are perfect for cleaning salon surfaces.

30. Jason can require the salon's stylists to use a ____ phenol solution for disinfecting metal implements.
    A. *5%*
    > A phenol is a caustic poison that can be safely and effectively used on metal implements if used according to the manufacturers' directions.

31. Because it is not effective for use in the salon environment, which of the following forms of alcohol can't the cleaning crew use?
    C. *Anopropryl*
    > The only types of alcohol that are sometimes used to disinfect implements in the salon are ethyl and isopropyl.

32. The cleaning crew's ability to sanitize is limited mainly to the practice of:
    A. *Washing tools and implements with detergent*
    > Sanitation is the lowest level of decontamination, and it involves significantly reducing the number of

pathogens or disease-producing organisms found on a surface such as a countertop.

33. Before immersing his implements into the disinfecting solution, Keith should:
    B. *Wash them with soap and water*
       Before putting soiled implements into a jar of disinfectant, Keith should sanitize them by washing them with soap and water.

34. To protect himself, Keith should wear _____ when working with disinfecting solution.
    D. *Gloves*
       Wearing gloves will protect his skin from becoming damaged, burned, or irritated by the chemical or liquid disinfectants he uses.

35. How should Keith mix the disinfecting solution?
    C. *According to the manufacturers' guidelines*
       All too often, professionals do not take the time to read the manufacturers' directions for how to mix and properly use disinfectants. Their unwillingness to do so may cause the mixture to be ineffectual and, therefore, they will not truly be as disinfecting as they should be.

36. How long should Keith's implements be immersed in the disinfecting solution?
    C. *As long as the directions recommend*
       Again, by not following the manufacturers' directions, persons using disinfectant solutions may not achieve the desired results if they remove implements from the solution too quickly, nor will they prevent any additional spread of disease by leaving their implements in a solution longer.

37. By reaching into the disinfecting solution and pulling out the implements without using tongs or a glove, what is Keith causing to happen to the disinfecting solution?
    A. *He is contaminating the solution*
       Keith is contaminating the disinfecting solution with whatever may be on his hands when he reaches into the disinfecting jar.

38. After the implements have been removed from the disinfecting solution, Keith should:

    B. *Place them in a clean, dry, disinfected container*

        Storing or placing implements or tools in anything but a clean, dry, disinfected container will only serve to infect them again.

Chapter 6

ANATOMY AND PHYSIOLOGY

CELLS

39. Malik's cells contain _____, a colorless, jelly-like substance in which food elements and water are present.
    B. *Protoplasm*
       Malik's cells and the cells of all living things are composed of protoplasm, which can be compared to the white of a raw egg.

40. The nucleus of Malik's cells play a vital role in:
    C. *Reproduction*
       The nucleus is a dense, active protoplasm found in the center of the cell, and it also plays a significant role in metabolism.

41. If Malik's cells are unable to repair themselves, the problem most likely lies in the cells':
    D. *Cytoplasm*
       The cytoplasm is all of the protoplasm of a cell except the nucleus, and is the watery fluid that contains the food material necessary for growth, reproduction, and self-repair.

42. The two phases of metabolism that Malik's cells undergo are:
    C. *Catabolism and anabolism*
       Anabolism is constructive metabolism; it is the act of building up larger molecules from smaller ones, and catabolism is the phase that involves breaking down of complex compounds within the cells into smaller ones.

TISSUES

43. The ____ tissue is responsible for supporting, protecting, and binding other tissues of the body together.
    C. *Connective*
        Some examples of connective tissue are bone, cartilage, ligaments, and fat or adipose tissue.

44. The tissue that carries food, waste, and hormones through the body is called:
    B. *Liquid*
        Liquid tissue such as blood and lymph carry vital elements and by-products through the body.

45. As an esthetician, Karen will be very interested in the epithelial tissue since it includes the:
    C. *Skin*
        The epithelial tissue is a protective covering on body surfaces such as the skin, mucous membranes, and the lining of the heart and digestive and respiratory organs.

46. When giving a facial massage, Karen will be coming into contact with the ____ system.
    D. *Muscular*
        Muscular tissue contracts and moves various parts of the body.

47. When a facial client realizes that she feels relaxed and calm as a result of Karen's facial manipulations, it will be because the ____ tissues are carrying those messages from the brain to the rest of the body.
    A. *Nerve*
        Nerve tissues not only carry messages to and from the brain but also are responsible for the coordination and control of all bodily functions.

ORGANS

48. The organs most useful to Richard in realizing that he is losing his hair are the:
     B. *Eyes*

     The eyes control our vision and make it possible to detect changes in ourselves, our surroundings, and in others.

49. When Richard is advised to massage his scalp, the doctor's intention is to increase Richard's blood circulation, which is a function of the:
     C. *Heart*

     The heart is responsible for all of the body's blood circulation, and by gently massaging his scalp, Richard is increasing the blood flow to that area.

50. Drinking plenty of clean water will allow Richard's body to eliminate waste products through the work of the:
     A. *Kidneys*

     The kidneys are responsible for eliminating excess water and waste from the body. Drinking plenty of water helps the kidneys have enough fluids to healthfully excrete waste and toxins when needed.

51. Supplying oxygen to the blood is the work of Richard's:
     C. *Lungs*

     Oxygen in the bloodstream helps the cells of the body perform their functions.

52. Using a cream or lotion will moisturize Richard's skin, which is responsible for:
     D. *Forming an external protective covering for the body*

     The skin is the organ that completely encloses and encases the body and all of its organs.

BODY SYSTEMS

53. While setting her hair, Billy notices that Mrs. Hammil's legs and ankles are swollen, which indicates that her _____ system is not working properly.

    D. *Excretory*

    The excretory system, which consists of the kidneys, liver, skin, intestines, and lungs, purifies the body by elimination of waste matter. Swollen legs indicate that the body is holding onto fluid instead of releasing it and the waste it contains.

54. Mrs. Boxing has difficulty controlling the position of her head during her service; she is experiencing difficulty with her:

    B. *Muscular system*

    The muscular system covers, shapes, and supports the skeleton tissue, and contracts and moves parts of the body.

55. During her perm, Mrs. Reyper sounds like she is having difficulty breathing. This is the work of the:

    D. *Respiratory system*

    The respiratory system enables the body to breathe by supplying oxygen and eliminating carbon dioxide as a waste product.

THE SKELETAL SYSTEM AND THE MUSCULAR SYSTEM

56. In the first part of the massage, Chris will begin at the crown and work her way down to the _____, which is above the nape.

    D. *Occipital bone*

    The occipital bone is the hindmost bone of the skull below the parietal bones, and it forms the back of the skull above the nape.

57. The muscle that Chris will be massaging when he works on Dennis' crown and occipital area is the:
    B. *Occipitalis*
        The occipitalis is in the back of the epicranius and is the muscle that draws the scalp backward.

58. The bone that forms Dennis' forehead is called the:
    B. *Frontal*
        The frontal bone is the large bone across the front, upper part of the face.

59. The muscle that allows Dennis to raise his eyebrows is the:
    A. *Frontalis*
        The frontalis is the anterior portion of the epicranius and it is the muscle of the scalp that raises the eyebrows, draws the scalp forward, and causes wrinkles across the forehead.

60. To relieve the tension at his temples, Chris will massage Dennis' _____ muscle.
    C. *Temporalis*
        The masseter and the temporalis muscles coordinate in opening and closing the mouth, and are sometimes referred to as the chewing muscles.

61. The bones that are Dennis' temples are the:
    C. *Temporal bones*
        The temporal bones are the bones that form the sides of the head in the ear region.

62. To relieve his neck aches, Chris suggests that Dennis sleep with a soft pillow supporting the seven bones of his:
    C. *Cervical vertebrae*
        The cervical vertebrae are the seven bones that form the top portion of the vertebral column located in the neck.

63. The muscles responsible for the movement of Dennis' neck and head is the:
    D. *Sternocleidomastoideus*
        This is the muscle of the neck that lowers and rotates the head.

64. When Betty massages Pam's fingers, the muscles that are responsible for separating the fingers are the:
    C. *Abductors*

    Abductors are the muscles that separate the fingers, and massaging them often provides relief from stiffness and fatigue.

65. While massaging Pam's fingers, Betty will be concentrating on massaging the bones of the:
    C. *Phalanges*

    The phalanges are the bones in the fingers consisting of three in each finger and two in the thumb.

66. Because of her work, she is in danger of having pain in her:
    B. *Carpus*

    The carpus is the wrist, a flexible joint composed of a group of eight small, irregular bones held together by ligaments.

67. In order to massage the palm of Pam's hand, Betty would come into contact with the:
    D. *Metacarpus*

    The metacarpus are bones of the palm of the hand; parts of the hand that contain five bones between the carpus and phalanges.

68. The muscles in the palm of Pam's hand that enable her to move her thumb toward her fingers is called the:
    B. *Opponent*

    These are the muscles in the palm that act to bring the thumb toward the fingers.

69. Betty finishes Pam's treatment by massaging her upper arm, also called the:
    B. *Humerus*

    The humerus is the uppermost and largest bone of the arm, extending from the elbow to the shoulder.

70. The muscle that allows Pam to rotate her palm outward is the:
    A. *Supinator*

    The supinator is the muscle that allows the forearm to rotate back and forth.

71. The muscle in Alma's forehead that is responsible for vertical wrinkles is the:
    D. *Corrugator*
    > This muscle is located beneath the frontalis and draws the eyebrow down as well.

72. The muscle between the cheek and upper and lower jaw that compresses the cheeks and gives Alma the appearance of high cheek bones is the:
    C. *Buccinator*
    > The buccinator is a thin, flat muscle of the cheek between the upper and lower jaw.

73. The muscle around Alma's eye socket that is toned so as to reduce the tiny wrinkles around her eyes is:
    A. *Orbicularis oculi*
    > This is a ring muscle of the eye socket that enables a person to close his eyes.

74. The muscle that causes wrinkles across the bridge of Alma's nose is the:
    B. *Procerus*
    > This muscle covers the bridge of the nose and lowers the eyebrows.

75. When she made her sarcastic comment about looking young, Alma employed her ____ muscle to lower her lower lip and draw it to one side.
    C. *Depressor labii inferioris*
    > This is the muscle surrounding the lower lip.

76. The muscle that would allow Alma to draw her lips into a pout is the:
    D. *Levator anguli oris*
    > This muscle raises the angle of the mouth and draws it inward.

THE NERVOUS SYSTEM

77. The system whose activities are responsible for Sean's thought processes about exercise is the:
    C. *Central nervous system*
       The central nervous system controls all consciousness and mental activities including all body movements and facial expressions.

78. When Sean realizes that he feels tired as a result of his workout, the realization is the ____system at work.
    B. *Peripheral*
       The function of this system is to carry messages to and from the central nervous system.

79. When Sean's heart rate becomes elevated, it is the response of the ____ system to the workout.
    A. *Autonomic*
       This system controls the involuntary muscles such as the heart, blood vessels, and glands.

80. The type of nerves that carry the sensation of Sean's leg cramps to the brain are the:
    A. *Afferent*
       These nerves carry messages from the sense organs to the brain.

81. The nerves that carry the message from his brain to his muscles, thus allowing Sean to pick up and move weights during his workout, are called:
    C. *Motor*
       These carry impulses from the brain to the muscles, and the transmitted impulses produce movement.

NERVES OF THE HEAD, FACE, AND NECK

82. When Mark pulls his ears away from his face and bends them downward, he is affecting the ____nerves.
    C. *Auriculotemporal*
       This nerve affects the external ear and skin above the temple up to the top of the skull.

83. When Anne puts her index finger on the tip of her nose and lifts it up slightly, she is affecting the ____ nerve.
    A. *Nasal*
       The nasal nerve affects the point and the lower side of the nose.

84. When Missy extends her lower lip and chin into a pout, she is affecting the ____ nerve.
    C. *Mental*
       This nerve affects the lower lip and chin.

85. When Matt raises his eyebrows as if he has just been shocked or surprised, he is affecting the ____ nerve.
    B. *Supraorbital*
       This nerve affects the skin of the forehead, scalp, eyebrow, and upper eyelid.

86. When Patsy pushes her lower lip and chin out from her face, she is affecting the ____ nerve.
    D. *Mandibular*
       This nerve affects the muscles of the chin and lower lip.

87. When Jo flashes a huge smile at the staff, she is affecting the ____ nerve.
    C. *Buccal*
       This nerve affects the muscles of the mouth.

THE CIRCULATORY SYSTEM

88. The circulatory system consists of John's ____, arteries, veins, and capillaries.
    B. *Heart*
       The heart is often referred to as the body's pump and is the cone-shaped muscle that keeps the blood moving throughout the body.

89. Why is John's heart pumping so rapidly?

A. *To supply blood to parts of the body so he can have the
    energy to move about*
    The more energy John needs, the faster his heart
    pumps to supply the proper amounts of blood and
    oxygen.

90. John's body is employing ____ circulation when it sends
     blood from the heart throughout the body and back to
     the heart again.
     C. *Systemic*
         There are two systems that attend to the body's
         circulation: pulmonary and systemic circulation.

91. John's heart is a:
     D. *Muscle*
         The heart is a cone-shaped muscle that keeps the
         blood moving throughout the body.

92. In order to purify it, John's heart will employ ____
     circulation to send his blood to his lungs.
     A. *Pulmonary*
         During pulmonary circulation, the blood is sent
         from the heart to the lungs for purification.

93. The thick-walled muscular tubes that carry oxygenated
     blood away from John's heart to the capillaries are called:
     C. *Arteries*
         Arteries carry the oxygenated blood to the other
         organs of the body. The largest of these is the aorta.

94. ____ are situated between the chambers of John's heart
     and they allow blood to flow in only one direction.
     A. *Valves*
         Valves open to allow blood flow and close again to
         prevent backflow of blood.

95. John has ____ , which are thin-walled blood vessels that
     are less elastic than arteries.
     D. *Veins*
         Veins carry blood containing waste from capillaries
         back to the heart.

96. John's ____ are minute, thin-walled blood vessels that

connect the smaller arteries to veins.
B. *Capillaries*
These bring nutrients to the cells and carry away waste materials.

97. John's red blood cells:
D. *Carry oxygen to the body's cells*
The red blood cells, also called red corpuscles, contain hemoglobin, a complex iron protein that gives blood its bright red color.

98. John's white blood cells:
B. *Destroy harmful germs*
White blood cells destroy disease-causing germs to keep the body healthy.

99. The plasma in John's blood is responsible for:
A. *Carrying food to cells*
The plasma carries food and secretions to the cells and carries away carbon dioxide.

100. Which of the following is NOT a function of John's lymph nodes?
A. *Provide waste to cells*
The lymph nodes carry nourishment from the blood to the cells, act as a defense against toxins, and remove waste from cells.

THE ENDOCRINE, DIGESTIVE, EXCRETORY, RESPIRATORY, AND INTEGUMENTARY SYSTEMS

101. The name of the system that affects the growth, development, and health of Joan's entire body is:
B. *Endocrine*
The endocrine system is made up of a group of specialized glands such as the pancreas that affect the general health of the body.

102. Joan's endocrine glands secrete ____ into her bloodstream,

which influence the well-being of her entire body.

A. *Hormones*

> Hormones, such as insulin and estrogen, stimulate functional activity and secretion in other parts of the body.

103. The hormone most directly responsible for Joan's hot flashes is:

C. *Estrogen*

> Estrogen is the hormone present in women and is responsible for menstrual and menopausal activity.

104. The ____, which is/are part of Joan's excretory system, is/are responsible for eliminating waste through perspiration.

C. *Skin*

> The skin purifies the body by eliminating waste through perspiration.

105. When she practices deep breathing exercises, Joan is employing her:

D. *Lungs*

> The lungs take in oxygen, then enable the body to exhale carbon dioxide.

106. The muscular wall that helps Joan control her breathing is the:

C. *Diaphragm*

> The diaphragm is a muscular wall that separates the thorax from the abdominal region and helps to control a person's breathing.

107. When Joan breathes in and oxygen is absorbed into her bloodstream, the process is called:

A. *Inhalation*

> The first part of the breathing cycle is inhalation.

108. When Joan breathes out and carbon dioxide is expelled from the body, the process is called:

C. *Exhalation*

> The second part of the breathing cycle is exhalation.

109. Joan's skin, oil and sweat glands, sensory receptors, hair, and nails all belong to which of the following body systems?
    B. *Integumentary*
        The integumentary system and its glands are of particular interest to the cosmetologist as they include the hair and nails.

110. The system responsible for changing Susan's burger into nutrients and waste is the:
    D. *Digestive*
        The digestive system is responsible for changing food into nutrients and waste.

111. Susan's ____ will be at work changing certain kinds of foods into a form that can be used by the body.
    C. *Enzymes*
        Digestive enzymes are responsible for changing certain types of foods into a form that can be used by the body for fuel.

112. If Susan eats her burger at 9:15 P.M., what time will it be when her body completes the entire digestive process?
    D. *6:15 A.M.*
        The entire digestive process takes approximately nine hours to complete.

113. The iced tea that Susan drinks will be metabolized by her kidneys and will leave her body in the form of:
    C. *Urine*
        Susan's kidneys will use the fluid to remove waste products in her body.

114. Any food that is not decomposed will be eliminated by Susan's:
    B. *Large intestine*
        It is the job of the large intestine to rid the body of decomposed and undigested food.

Chapter 7

BASICS OF CHEMISTRY AND ELECTRICITY

CHEMISTRY

115. The gasoline that Jack put into his car is considered to be:
    B. *Organic*
        Gas is considered organic because it is manufactured from natural gas and oil, which are the remains of plants and animals that died millions of years ago.

116. Jack's gasoline is classified as it is because it contains:
    B. *Carbon*
        Any substance that contains carbon is considered to be organic.

117. Jack's car, made of metal and steel, is considered:
    D. *Inorganic*
        Since Jack's car is made of metal, a nonliving thing, it is considered to be inorganic.

118. The bottle of water that Jack bought is an example of:
    B. *Matter*
        Matter is any substance that takes up space, and can be a liquid, solid, or gas.

119. Jack's pack of chewing gum exists in what form?
    D. *Solid*
        The pack of chewing gum Jack bought is a solid because it occupies space and is tangible.

120. The haircolor that Jack will apply to Mr. Ramirez is considered to be:
    A. *An organic substance*
        Haircolor is an organic substance because it is made from either a natural or synthetic source of organic compound.

121. The permanent wave solution that Jack will apply to Ms. Crepa is considered to be:
   A. *An organic substance*
      Perm wave solution is an organic substance because it is made from either a natural or synthetic source of organic compound.

122. Ms. Crepa's steam facial is an example of water in what form?
   C. *Gas*
      Steam is considered to be a gas because it does not have definite shape or volume.

123. When Jack evaluates Mr. Ramirez's natural hair color level, he is determining its:
   C. *Physical properties*
      Physical properties are those things that can be determined without a chemical reaction and don't cause a chemical change in the substance.

124. When Jack assesses the change in curl from before Ms. Crepa's perm to after it, he is assessing its:
   A. *Chemical properties*
      A chemical property can only be observed through a chemical change in the original substance such as a permanently curled section of hair.

125. When Mr. Ramirez's hair is cut, the change is considered to be:
   B. *Physical*
      It's a physical change because it did not require chemical reaction to change the substance.

126. When Mr. Ramirez's hair is colored, the change is considered to be:
   A. *Chemical*
      The haircolor is considered a chemical change because it did require a chemical reaction to change the substance.

PURE SUBSTANCES AND PHYSICAL MIXTURES

127. The water that Sierra uses to rinse her tools is an example of a:
   A. *Chemical compound*
      Water is a chemical compound because it is composed of two different atoms from two elements that combine to create a substance that is totally different from the elements with which it was made.

128. The foundation that Sierra used on Nancy's face during the makeup application is an example of a:
   B. *Physical compound*
      The foundation is a physical compound because despite the fact that the two elements were mixed together to form something else, they still held onto their original properties.

129. When Sierra blended the powder and the water for application to Nancy's skin, she made a:
   C. *Solution*
      The powder and water were a blended solution of two or more solids, liquids, or gaseous substances.

130. The powder that Sierra blended into the water is considered to be a:
   C. *Solute*
      A solute is the matter that is dissolved into a solvent such as the powder was when blended into the water.

131. The liquid into which Sierra blended the powder is considered to be a:
   A. *Solvent*
      A solvent, such as water, is the substance that dissolves another substance to form a solution with chemical change in the composition.

132. The fact that the water and powder mixed together without separating implies that they are:
   B. *Miscible*
      Miscible substances are those that can be mixed, in any proportion, without separating.

133. Since the foundation that Sierra used had to be shaken every time it was used because the two compounds kept separating, it is an example of a/an ____ substance.
    D. *Immiscible*
        An immiscible substance is one that is not capable of being mixed such as water and oil.

134. The facial scrub that Sierra applied to Nancy's skin is an example of a ____ because it contains solid particles distributed throughout a liquid form.
    D. *Suspension*
        A suspension is a state in which solid particles are distributed throughout a liquid medium.

135. The hair conditioner that was applied to Nancy's hair is an example of an:
    D. *Oil-in-water emulsion*
        An oil-in-water emulsion is one in which oil droplets are suspended in a water base such as in the case of a conditioner.

136. The cold cream that was applied to Nancy's skin is an example of a:
    A. *Water-in-oil emulsion*
        A water-in-oil emulsion is one in which water droplets are suspended in an oil base such as in the case of a cold cream.

COMMON PRODUCT INGREDIENTS

137. Mike's colleagues like using an alcohol that evaporates quickly for their needs in the salon. This type of alcohol is called:
    C. *Volatile*
        A volatile alcohol is useful in the salon to cleanse surfaces and it does evaporate quickly.

138. Which of the items on the list above is a form of ammonia?
     D. *Chemical hair relaxer*
         Ammonia is a form of colorless gas that is used to raise the pH level such as a chemical relaxing service.

139. Which of the items on the list above contain glycerin?
     C. *Hand cream*
         Glycerin is a sweet, colorless, oily substance formed by the decomposition of oils, fats, or fatty acids.

140. Which of the items on the list above contain silicones?
     C. *Sunblock*
         A silicone is a special type of oil used in hair conditioners and as a water-resistant lubricant for the skin.

141. Which of the items on the list above contain volatile organic compounds (VOCs)?
     A. *Hairspray*
         Volatile organic compounds are two or more elements combined chemically that contain carbon and evaporate quickly.

POTENTIAL HYDROGEN (PH)

142. When shampooing Barbra's hair, Marco will use water, which has a pH of:
     C. *7*
         Water has a pH of 7, which means that it is neither acidic nor alkaline.

143. The pH of the water Marco will use is considered to be:
     D. *Neutral*
         Water is considered neutral because it is in the middle of the scale, neither acidic nor alkaline.

144. The pH of Barbra's hair and skin is:
     B. *5*
         Hair and skin has a pH of 5.

145. The pH of Barbra's hair and skin is considered to be:
   A. *Acidic*
       A pH of 5 indicates that a substance is acidic.

146. Plain water is ____ than Barbara's hair and skin.
   D. *100 times more alkaline*
       Since the pH scale is a logarithmic scale, a change
       of one number indicates a ten-fold change, so a
       change of two whole numbers indicates a change of
       10 times 10, or 100 times.

147. The chemical hair relaxer treatment that Mandy will
    receive will have a pH that indicates it is:
   B. *Alkaline*
       All alkalis have a pH of above 7.

148. An alkaline pH is useful in straightening Mandy's hair
    because it will:
   D. *Soften and swell the hair*
       The alkaline pH softens and swells the hair, and
       allows the stylist to easily reform the hair into a shape
       that the client desires, in this case, to straighten the
       hair.

149. When Marco performs his perm service later in the day
    for Renee, the perm will have a pH that indicates it is an:
   A. *Acidic*
       An acidic pH is one that is below 7.

150. An acidic pH is useful in perm waving hair because it will
    ____ Renee's hair.
   A. *Harden and contract*
       To have the hair harden and contract around a
       perm rod and take on the shape of that rod is the
       purpose of a permanent wave.

151. After relaxing Mandy's hair, Marco will use a normalizing
    lotion that will neutralize the relaxer by creating a:
   C. *Acid-alkaline reaction*
       An acid-alkaline reaction is one in which an equal
       part of acid is added to an equal amount of alkaline
       and they neutralize each other, forming water.

152. When Marco's haircolor client, Andrea, has her service, he will witness a/an:

D. *Oxidation-reduction reaction*

An oxidation-reduction reaction is responsible for the chemical changes created by combining an element or compound with oxygen.

153. If, when perming Renee's hair, an element is combined with oxygen, ____ will be produced.

C. *Heat*

The heat is produced by the addition of oxygen to an element or compound in the oxidation process.

154. If heat is released during her perm, Renee's hair is experiencing an ____ reaction.

C. *Exothermic*

Chemical reactions that are characterized by the release of heat are called exothermic. The heat is produced by an oxidation reaction.

ELECTRICITY

155. Carlene's car employs a constant, even-flowing current, generated by a battery, which is called:

C. *Direct current*

Carlene's car battery creates a constant current that travels in one direction only and produces a chemical reaction; this process is called direct current.

156. The form of energy Carlene was fumbling to activate when she entered the salon is called:

B. *Electricity*

Electricity is a form of energy that when in motion, exhibits magnetic, chemical, or thermal effects.

157. An _____ is what accounts for the lights coming on when Carlene flipped the switch.

C. *Electric current*

An electric current is the flow of electricity along a conductor.

158. Supporting the switch that Carlene turned on is a/an ____, which conducts electricity.
    C. *Conductor*
        A conductor is any substance, material, or medium that can conduct electricity.

159. Carlene's silk blouse is a:
    B. *Nonconductor*
        A nonconductor is any substance, material, or medium that cannot easily conduct electricity such as Carlene's blouse.

160. When Carlene plugs her travel curling iron into the wall outlet, she is using an apparatus known as a:
    B. *Converter*
        A converter is an apparatus that changes direct current to alternating current.

161. When Carlene plugs her straight irons into the wall outlet, she is using:
    D. *Alternating current*
        Alternating current is rapid and interrupted current, flowing first in one direction and then in the opposite direction.

162. Carlene's cordless electric clippers are an example of a:
    A. *Rectifier*
        A rectifier is an apparatus that changes alternating current to direct current.

ELECTRICAL MEASUREMENTS

163. Martin learns that normal wall sockets that power hair dryers and curling irons are ____ volts.
    A. *110*
        A volt is a unit that measures the pressure or force that pushes the flow of electrons forward through a conductor. The normal rate for voltage power blow-dryers and other electrical apparatuses used in the salon are 110.

164. Outlets that can accommodate the correct amount of power for washing machines and dryers are _____ volts.
     B. *220*
          Since the work of a large appliance such as a washing machine or air conditioner requires more pressure, more force, and more power, these apparatuses require a 220 voltage.

165. Andy explains that, due to its _____ rating, a hair dryer cord must be twice as thick as an appliance rated lower in order to avoid overheating and starting a fire.
     B. *Amp*
          An amp (or ampere) is the unit that measures the strength of an electric current.

166. To create an atmosphere that is relaxing in the facial room, Martin will use a 40- _____ bulb.
     D. *Watt*
          A watt is a measurement of how much electricity is being used in a second.

167. Martin's 2,000-watt blow-dryer will use _____ watts of energy per second.
     D. *2,000*
          Each electrical implement or apparatus will be labeled with how many watts it uses so you can be aware of its electrical needs.

168. If a fuse gets too hot and melts, Martin will know that:
     D. *An excessive amount of current was prevented from passing through the circuit*
          The fuse melted when the wire became too hot and overloaded the circuit with too much current from too many appliances or from faulty equipment.

169. If too many appliances are operating on the same circuit and they all suddenly stop working, Martin will know that the _____ has shut off to protect the salon from a dangerous situation.
     C. *Circuit breaker*
          A circuit breaker is a switch that automatically shuts off or interrupts electric current at the first indication of overload.

ELECTROTHERAPY

170. Gale has prepared an electrode which is an ____ for use in treating Karen.
    A. *Applicator*
        An applicator made of carbon, glass, or metal is used for directing the electric current from the machine to the client's skin.

171. Gale determines that the positive electrode she will use, called the ____ , is red.
    C. *Anode*
        The anode is usually red and it will have a plus sign on it, indicating that it is a positive electrode.

172. The first modality Gale will use is called ____ current, which is a constant and direct current.
    B. *Galvanic*
        Galvanic current is used as a constant and direct current that produces chemical changes when it passes through the tissues and fluids of the body.

173. If Gale wants to force acidic substances into Karen's skin, she must use:
    B. *Cataphoresis*
        Cataphoresis forces acidic substances into deeper tissues using galvanic current from the positive toward the negative pole.

174. If Gale wants to force liquid into Karen's tissues, she must use:
    C. *Anaphoresis*
        Anaphoresis is the process of forcing liquids into the tissues from the negative toward the positive pole.

175. If Gale wants to introduce water-soluble products into Karen's skin, she must use:
    A. *Iontophoresis*
        Iontophoresis is the process of introducing water-soluble products into the skin with the use of electric current such as the use of positive and negative poles of a galvanic machine.

176. The process Gale will use to soften and emulsify the trapped oil deposits and blackheads on Karen's nose is called:
D. *Disincrustation*
This process is used to remove grease deposits and blackheads in hair follicles; the process is also frequently used for clients with acne and milia.

177. In order to improve Karen's muscle tone, Gale will employ ____ current.
D. *Faradic*
Faradic current is an alternating and interrupted current that produces a mechanical reaction without a chemical effect.

178. In order to calm Karen's nerves, Gale will employ ____ current.
C. *Sinusoidal*
Sinusoidal current is an alternating current that produces mechanical contractions that tone the muscles and soothe nerves.

179. To relieve Karen of congestion, Gale will employ ____ current.
A. *Tesla high-frequency*
Tesla high-frequency is a thermal current with a high rate of vibration, commonly called violet rays, that is used both for scalp and facial treatments. Its effects can be either stimulating or soothing.

180. To increase glandular activity, Gale may use a ____ on Karen.
C. *Vibrator*
A vibrator is used in massage to produce a mechanical succession of manipulations.

LIGHT THERAPY

181. The bright sunlight that Debbie experienced while running her errands is called:
D. *Visible light*
Visible light is electromagnetic radiation that we can see.

182. Since Debbie has a slight tan, she has been exposed to:
    A. *UV rays*
        UV rays make up 5 percent of natural sunlight and
        are the least penetrating of all sun rays. They produce
        chemical effects and kill germs.

183. To offer tanning services in the salon, Debbie and Larry
    must make sure that the UV rays are applied ____ inches
    from a light source.
    C. *30 to 36*
        The application of UV rays can be beneficial if done
        cautiously and with care; applied 30 to 36 inches
        away from the light source is the recommended
        distance for safety.

184. Once the light source is correctly placed, it is safe, and
    Debbie and Larry's clients can have their first session
    under the light source. The first session should last ____
    minutes.
    B. *2 to 3*
        The therapy should begin at 2 to 3 minutes of
        exposure time and can be increased gradually to 7 to 8
        minutes of exposure time.

185. Beth explains that infrared rays:
    C. *Penetrate the deepest*
        Infrared rays make up 60 percent of natural
        sunlight, have long wavelengths, and produce the
        most heat.

186. Beth explains that using ____ light is helpful for killing
    germs and should be used on bare skin.
    C. *Blue*
        Blue light should only be used on oily, bare skin; it
        contains few heat rays, is the least penetrating, and
        has some germicidal and chemical benefits.

187. When Larry asks her about dry skin, Beth recommends
    using ____ light in combination with oils and creams.
    D. *Red*
        Red light penetrates the deepest and produces the
        most heat.

Part III Hair Care

CHAPTER 8

PROPERTIES OF THE HAIR AND SCALP

STRUCTURE AND CHEMICAL COMPOSITION OF THE HAIR

1. When Mrs. Brand has her hair colored or permed, the chemical solution affects which layer of the hair shaft?
    B. *Cuticle*
        The cuticle is the outermost layer of the hair and it consists of a single layer of transparent, scale-like cells that overlap like shingles on a roof.

2. If Mrs. Brand's hair looks and feels dry and rough, it is most likely a result of:
    D. *Swelling of the cuticle layer of the hair*
        A healthy, compact cuticle layer is the hair's primary defense against damage. When a chemical such as haircolor or perm solution is administered to the hair, it causes the cuticle to swell to complete its action. Over time, the swollen cuticle can have the appearance of dry, rough hair.

3. In order for her permanent hair color and waving solution to actually change the hair's look, which layer of Mrs. Brand's hair must be affected?
    C. *Cortex*
        The cortex, the middle layer of the hair, is where all of the hair's melanin pigment is contained. During a

permanent haircolor service, the color molecules must penetrate the cortex in order to permanently change the hair's color.

4. The appearance of Mrs. Brand's hair indicates that:
   C. *The cuticle has been opened many times*
   > The dry, rough texture of Mrs. Brand's hair indicates that the cuticle has probably been opened repeatedly as a result of haircoloring and other chemical services.

5. Based on the information you have on Mrs. Brand, it is very likely that her hair is missing a:
   D. *Medulla*
   > The medulla is the innermost layer of the hair, and it is common for people with fine hair or naturally blond hair to entirely lack a medulla.

6. Mrs. Brand's hair is made up of ____ protein.
   C. *91%*
   > All hair is made up of 91 percent keratin protein, which is made up of long chains of amino acids. These, in turn, are made up of elements.

7. When Mrs. Brand's hair is colored or permed, the bonds that are broken are called:
   D. *Disulfide bonds*
   > A disulfide bond is a chemical side bond that can only be broken by the action of a chemical hair relaxer or permanent wave solution.

8. When Mrs. Brand's hair is wet set, the bonds that are broken are called:
   B. *Hydrogen bonds*
   > A hydrogen bond is a physical side bond that is easily broken by water or heat, thus allowing for Mrs. Brand's hair to curl when wet set.

9. When Mrs. Brand's hair is permed, the bonds that are broken are called:
   C. *Salt bonds*
   > Salt bonds are physical side bonds that are broken by changes in pH such as an acidic or alkaline solution.

10. Mrs. Brand's natural blond hair is a result of the ____ in her hair's cortex.
    C. *Pheomelanin*
    > Pheomelanin provides natural hair colors ranging from red and ginger to yellow/blond tones. Natural hair color is the result of the ratio of eumelanin to pheomelanin, along with the total number and size of pigment granules.

HAIR ANALYSIS AND GROWTH

11. In determining the texture of Marlene's hair, John notes that it is:
    D. *Coarse*
    > Coarse hair has the largest diameter, is stronger than fine hair, and has a strong structure.

12. Based on his diagnosis, Marlene's hair diameter and structure are characterized as:
    C. *Large and coarse*
    > Marlene has coarse hair, which indicates that her hair is characterized as being large and strong.

13. John must be aware of Marlene's hair texture because it may affect the outcome of:
    B. *The haircolor service*
    > Coarse hair usually requires more processing time than medium or fine hair and may also be more resistant to processing. John must know this in order to plan the service properly.

14. Based on what he felt when he touched her head, John noted that Marlene's hair density is:
    D. *High*
    > A high hair density indicates that a person has many hairs on her head, but it has no real relation to a person's hair texture.

15. Marlene's hair density indicates that she has:
    D. *A lot of hairs per square inch on her head*

    Marlene has very dense hair, which indicates that regardless of her hair texture, she has many hairs on her head.

16. Based on Marlene's hair color, how many hairs is she likely to carry on her head?
    B. *110,000*

    Generally, people with brown hair have approximately 110,000 hairs on their head at any given time.

17. Based on John's diagnosis of Marlene's hair, what is her hair's porosity likely to be?
    A. *Low*

    Because of her hair's texture and condition, John realizes that Marlene's hair has low porosity, which means that it is considered resistant.

18. Chemical services performed on hair with Marlene's porosity require a/an:
    C. *Alkaline solution*

    John will need to use an alkaline solution on Marlene's hair because it will be necessary to sufficiently open the cuticle to allow for uniform saturation and processing.

19. Based on John's observations, Marlene's hair elasticity would be categorized as:
    D. *Normal*

    Marlene's hair elasticity is normal because when it is stretched, it is able to return to its normal position. Hair with normal elasticity can stretch up to 50 percent of its original length and return without breaking.

20. The growth pattern that is evident on the back of Marlene's head is called a:
    B. *Whorl*

    A whorl is hair that forms a circular pattern and is normally found on a person's crown.

21. John must remember Marlene's growth pattern, especially when:

    D. *Cutting her hair*

    John will need to be aware of Marlene's growth pattern, then make plans to compensate for the pattern when cutting her hair to make sure not to cut the hair too short and to have an even, finished look.

22. What type of hair and scalp condition does Marlene have?

    D. *Oily hair and scalp*

    Based on the feel of the hair—slick and greasy—John can determine that Marlene has overactive sebaceous glands that render the scalp and hair oily.

HAIR LOSS

23. As she services Albert and learns about his hair loss, Bonnie realizes that his type of hair loss is categorized as:

    A. *Androgenic alopecia*

    Androgenic alopecia is hair loss as a result of genetics, age, and hormonal changes that cause miniaturization of terminal hair.

24. The cause of Albert's hair loss is likely to be his:

    B. *Age*

    Based on his age and the condition of his hair and scalp, which otherwise appear to be healthy, Bonnie can safely assume his hair loss is simply a result of aging.

25. Anna's hair loss is categorized as:

    D. *Postpartum alopecia*

    Postpartum alopecia is temporary hair loss as a result of pregnancy.

26. Anna's hair loss is usually:
    B. *Temporary with hair growth returning to normal within a year*
       Usually, a woman who experiences hair loss during pregnancy can expect her hair growth cycle to return to normal within a year after delivery.

27. Martin's type of hair loss is called:
    C. *Alopecia areata*
       Alopecia areata is characterized by the sudden loss of hair in round patches, either on the scalp or on other areas of the body.

28. Martin's hair loss is caused by:
    C. *An unpredictable autoimmune skin disease*
       Alopecia areata is caused by the person's own hair follicles mistakenly attacked by the person's own immune system with white blood cells stopping the hair growth phase.

DISORDERS OF THE HAIR AND SCALP

29. The technical term for Mrs. Hines' gray hair is:
    A. *Canities*
       Canities is the technical term for gray hair and is caused by the loss of the hair's natural melanin pigment.

30. The technical term for Mrs. Hines' striped hair is:
    D. *Ringed hair*
       Ringed hair is a variety of canities and is characterized by alternating bands of gray and pigmented hair throughout the length of the strand.

31. The dark hair on Sandra's upper lip is a result of:
    B. *Hirsuties*
       Hirsuties is a condition characterized by abnormal hair growth.

32. The technical term for Jan's split ends is:
     D. *Trichoptilosis*
         Trichoptilosis is usually caused by hair damage, and
         may be treated by deep conditioning services or by
         simply trimming off the affected hair.

33. The technical term for Joe's knotted and breaking hair is:
     B. *Trichorrhexis nodosa*
         Trichorrhexis nodosa is characterized by brittleness
         and the formation of nodular swellings along the hair
         shaft.

34. The small white flakes Joe finds when brushing or
     combing his hair are called:
     D. *Pitryasis*
         Pitryasis is the medical term for dandruff, the small
         white scales that appear on the scalp and in the hair.

35. The technical term for head lice is:
     C. *Pediculosis capitis*
         Head lice are animal parasites that infest the hair
         and scalp and cause itching and infection.

CHAPTER 9

PRINCIPLES OF HAIR DESIGN

PHILOSOPHY OF DESIGN AND ELEMENTS OF HAIR DESIGN

36. Andie's excitement over what she learned at the hair show and her desire to try out some of the techniques is considered to be:
    A. *Inspiration*
       Inspiration is the stimulus that motivates action and creativity. Andie was inspired by the styles she saw at the hair show to go home and try out what she learned.

37. When designing a style for hair that forces the eye to look up and down, Andie is creating a hairstyle with:
    B. *Vertical lines*
       Vertical lines in a style make it appear longer and narrower as the eye follows the lines up and down.

38. Cathy, one of Andie's clients, is a single mom with three children who is looking for a very simple hairstyle that requires the least amount of care, so she must consider a:
    A. *Single line hairstyle*
       Since the single line hairstyle is the simplest to care for, it is best worn by someone who wants an easy-to-wear and easy-to-care for look.

39. To create the illusion of a more slender face for her client Joan, Andie could use haircolor that is a:
    C. *Dark color*
       Dark colors cause the face to look smaller or thinner. To create the illusion of a more slender face, Andie should use a dark color where appropriate.

40. To create a hairstyle that reflects the most light for her client, Meredith, Andie should consider a style with a ____ wave pattern.
    D. *Straight*
       Curly hair, because of its movement and curl, tends to cut up the ability of the hair to reflect light. Straight hair, on the other hand, does not chop up the light and, therefore, has the appearance of super shine.

PRINCIPLES OF HAIR DESIGN, AND CREATING HARMONY BETWEEN HAIRSTYLE AND FACIAL STRUCTURE

41. Based on Kim's description of her face, she has a/an ____ face shape.
    C. *Round*
       A round face type is characterized as being round at the hairline and chin line, with a wide face.

42. To help a round face shape appear longer and thinner, the best hairstyle is one that:
    D. *Creates volume at the top and is close at the sides*
       The best style for a round face shape is one that creates volume at the top but is close at the sides, thus creating the appearance of a long, narrow line.

43. To minimize the appearance of Kim's forehead, Courtney should style her hair:
    D. *Forward over the sides of the forehead*
       By styling Kim's hair forward over the sides of the forehead, Courtney can hide the wideness of the forehead while still maintaining the illusion of a narrow line down the middle of the face.

44. To combat her close-set eyes, Kim's hair should be:
    A. *Directed back and away from the temples*
       Directing the hair back and away from the temples will open up the eye area and make them appear further apart.

45. What type of part is best for a face with a wide flat nose?
    C. *Center part*
        A center part gives the appearance of length.

46. To bring more definition to Kim's jawline, which type of line should be used?
    C. *Straight*
        A straight line at the chin draws attention to that area and away from the center of the face.

47. When restyling Kim's hair, Courtney will need to make sure her wavy hair is _____ at the temple area and _____ at the top.
    A. *Close, high*
        To give the round face a more slender appearance, Courtney will need to make sure the hair is close at the temples to eliminate width and high at the top to give the illusion of an elongated shape.

Chapter 10

SHAMPOOING, RINSING, AND CONDITIONING

UNDERSTANDING SHAMPOO AND CONDITIONERS

48. Barton is a 15-year-old client of the salon who frequently uses a lot of thick styling glue to get his hair into long spikes. He notices that his hair sometimes feels gooey even after shampooing. Alexia recommends a/an _____ shampoo for him.

   D. *Clarifying*

   Because of all of the product Barton uses on his hair and its formula of ingredients, he is experiencing a buildup of product; that's what feels gooey to him. A clarifying shampoo contains an acidic ingredient such as cider vinegar that is helpful in cutting through product buildup that can flatten the hair or make it appear less shiny and healthy.

49. Mrs. Kames is a long time haircolor client and needs a shampoo that will enable her to keep her color looking fresh between retouch visits. She should try a/an _____ shampoo.

   B. *Color-enhancing*

   A color-enhancing shampoo cleanses the hair and adds the color base back to the hair, acting like a temporary color. This is very useful to clients who want to keep the original tone of their color looking fresh.

50. Alexia usually suggests a client with _____ hair purchase a moisturizing shampoo.

   B. *Permed*

   A client, whose hair may be dry or damaged due to chemicals used in the salon, can greatly benefit from a moisturizing shampoo, which will make the hair feel smooth and shiny.

51. For Norman's oily scalp, Alexia suggests a ____ shampoo.
    A. *Balancing*
       A balancing shampoo is made especially for oily hair and scalp, and will wash away excess oiliness without drying the scalp excessively.

52. For Joyce, who washes, blow-dries, and hot curls her hair every day, Alexia recommends a ____ conditioner.
    C. *Leave-in*
       For someone who mechanically damages her hair as much as Joyce does with her regime each day, a leave-in conditioner, one that is applied and not rinsed out, is ideal to moisturize and protect the hair from additional damage.

53. For Janice, who has a full head of bleached hair, Alexia recommends an in-salon conditioning service and a ____ conditioner for at-home use.
    B. *Treatment*
       For hair such as Janice's that is extremely damaged and dry, a treatment or repair conditioning treatment is excellent. These conditioners are left on the hair for up to 20 minutes, sometimes employ heat, and generally penetrate the cuticle by restoring protein and conditioners to the dry hair.

Chapter 11

HAIRCUTTING

BASIC PRINCIPLES OF HAIRCUTTING

54. Erin, Johnny's first customer, loves to wear an old haircutting favorite: the wedge. Johnny will use her occipital bone as his ____ for the entire cut.
    B. *Reference point*
        A reference point is a point on the head that marks where the surface of the head changes and is used by haircutters to establish design lines that are proportionate to the head.

55. When cutting a client's hair for the first time, Johnny is careful to observe the ____ for unusual growth patterns such as cowlicks.
    D. *Crown*
        The crown is the area between the apex and the back of the parietal ridge, usually the site of cowlicks and whorls.

56. When cutting long hair along the face to connect the bangs and the nape, Johnny often cuts a ____ line.
    D. *Diagonal*
        Diagonal lines are used to connect two varying lengths, and are cut in a slanting or sloping direction.

57. When Johnny cuts Marianne's hair into a one-length bob, he uses ____ degrees of elevation.
    A. *0*
        Zero degrees of elevation give a straight, blunt, one-length haircut.

58. Marianne's bob will be uniform if Johnny makes sure to continuously use his initial ____ guideline when cutting.
     A. *Stationary*
         A stationary guideline does not move. To cut the hair, all of the subsections are brought to the guide and cut at that elevation.

59. Darla has very long hair that she wants to be layered. To keep her long at the nape, Johnny cuts it by ____ the hair.
     B. *Overdirecting*
         Overdirection occurs by combing the hair away from its natural falling position, thus allowing a cutter to keep certain areas of hair significantly longer than other areas while still achieving a blended looking haircut.

CLIENT CONSULTATION AND TOOLS

60. Lucy asks Pat what he thinks about her having her hair cut really short so it can just lay flat against her face. Pat explains that a cut like that will cause her hair to:
     B. *Stand up away from the scalp*
         Thick, coarse hair that is cut too short will not lie flat; rather, because the weight will be taken away from the strand, it will spring up and stick out.

61. Which tool should Pat NOT use when cutting Lucy's hair?
     C. *Razor*
         Since a razor gives a soft finish to hair ends, using a razor on Lucy's thick and course hair will serve to lighten the ends even more and further cause her hair to stand up on end.

62. Frank likes to wear his hair short around the bottom and sides and fuller on top with a messy look. To achieve this, Pat will need to use ____ on the top.
     D. *Thinning shears*
         Wearing hair "messy" means that the hair will need to be cut into different lengths to achieve the messy look, where the shorter hairs hold up the longer hairs.

This is beautifully achieved with the use of a thinning shear.

63. To get a clean line at the nape, Pat will employ a/an:
   D. *Edger*
   > An edger is a smaller version of a clipper and is mainly used to clean the nape line on very short cuts.

64. To create the look of thicker hair, Pat needs to create _____ in Susan's style.
   B. *Weight*
   > In order to create the illusion of thicker hair, Pat will need to find a way to create weight. This can be done by cutting the hair at a 0-degree elevation.

65. The best cut for Susan's hair is the:
   B. *Blunt cut*
   > A blunt cut, or a zero elevation cut, builds weight lines on the head form and gives the illusion of thicker hair.

66. The best cutting tool for Pat to use on Susan's hair is:
   B. *Haircutting shears*
   > Since Pat wants to get an exacting, blunt cut for Susan's one-length style, the best tool he can use is simple haircutting shears.

67. The type of comb that Pat will use for each of his haircuts will be the:
   D. *Styling comb*
   > A styling or cutting comb is between six and eight inches long and is considered an all-purpose comb, used for most cutting procedures.

CUTTING CURLY HAIR

68. To give Jen the trim she wants, Manny will need to:
   B. *Cut it straight across the bottom with no tension at all*
   > Pulling curly hair taut when cutting will cause it to be much shorter when it dries, so to preserve its length, Manny will want to cut it without tension.

69. To achieve the appearance of having cut Jen's hair one inch, Manny will actually need to cut off about:
B. $^1/_4$ *inch*
> The rule of thumb for cutting curly hair is that for every $^1/_4$ inch that's cut, the hair will shrink by about one inch.

70. Cutting one inch of hair will make Jen's finished style appear ____ when it is dry.
C. *Shorter*
> Cutting Jen's hair a full inch will make her hair appear much shorter than she wants it to be.

71. When Manny begins cutting Sandy's hair, he must be aware that her curly hair will need to be elevated ____ to achieve the desired look.
C. *Less*
> Since Sandy wants her hair to be layered, Manny will need to employ some elevation in his cutting technique; however, it should be less elevation when working with curly hair than with straight hair cut into the same style.

72. To give Sandy's hair the chunky look she desires, he will need to texturize her hair using the ____ technique.
C. *Notching*
> Notching is a more aggressive version of point cutting and delivers a chunky look to the hair.

73. To give Renee the mid-length style she desires, Manny will need to cut the hair at a ____ -degree angle all around the head.
B. *45*
> Using a 45-degree angle will give Renee the mid-length layered look she is after.

74. To remove bulk and to add movement to Renee's cut, Manny will use a technique called:
D. *Slicing*
> Slicing is a great technique for removing bulk and adding movement throughout the lengths of the hair.

Chapter 12

HAIRSTYLING

WET HAIRSTYLING BASICS, FINGER WAVING, PIN CURLS, ROLLER CURLS, AND COMB-OUT TECHNIQUES

75. The list of supplies Gayle will need to have handy for styling the two characters include:
    D. *Clips, combs, and rollers*
    > Creating these two beautifully coifed styles will require an artistic eye and wet set styling tools such as clips, combs, and rollers.

76. In terms of styling aids, Gayle will need to purchase:
    A. *Setting lotion, styling lotion, and hairspray*
    > These are the exact types of wet goods products that are useful in wet setting hair.

77. To achieve the close-to-the-head waves the director wants Esther to wear, Gayle will need to create:
    C. *A finger wave*
    > A finger wave, with its perfectly aligned curl formations that lay flat against the head, is the perfect technique to achieve this look.

78. To ensure that Esther's hair lays appropriately for the style, Gayle should use:
    C. *Her natural part*
    > Using her natural part ensures that the hair will lie flat instead of fighting with a part line that forces the hair to lay in a direction that it doesn't want to lay in.

79. The best type of comb for Gayle to use when creating Esther's style is a:
    B. *Styling comb*
    > A styling comb is perfectly balanced and is the correct comb for Gayle to use when forming Esther's style.

80. When Gayle completes styling Esther's hair, it should look like a continuous:
    C. S
    Finger waves that are done correctly should look like one continuous S shape all over the head, and each ridge should be the exact same size and shape as the one before it.

81. How should Gayle dry Esther's hair prior to combing it out?
    D. With a hooded dryer
    To dry Esther's hair, Gayle should use a hair net to protect the style from excessive blowing, then put her under a hooded dryer until the style is completely dry.

82. To create Johanna's style, Gayle will use:
    D. A hooded dryer, rollers, and pin curls
    To get the kind of volume and hold needed for this role, Gayle will use a wet set.

83. To create the most volume she can on the top of Johanna's head, Gayle will place:
    A. Rollers on base
    By rolling the hair on the roller and placing it directly on top of its base, Gayle ensures that her curl will have the greatest volume and mobility.

84. In order for Johanna's hair to sweep forward at her temples, Gayle will place pin curls into a/an ____ shaping.
    C. C
    The C shaping will first sweep the hair at the temple area back off the face and then forward again, onto the face.

85. In order to get a tight, long-lasting curl without too much mobility, Gayle will use:
    A. No stem pin curls
    The no stem pin curl is placed directly on the base of the curl and delivers a tight, firm, long-lasting curl with little mobility.

86. To achieve a smooth, directed shape, Gayle will need to use a/an ____base pin curl at the temple area of Johanna's style.
    C. *Arc*
        Arc based pin curls are carved out of a base shaping, give good direction, and are used around the hairline.

87. When combing out the finished style, Gayle will certainly need to ____the hair on the top of Johanna's head to achieve the height she desires and to ensure the shape lasts as long as needed.
    B. *Back comb*
        Back combing or teasing involves combing small sections of hair from the ends to the base, causing shorter hair to mat at the base and form a cushion or base.

BLOW-DRY STYLING AND TOOLS

88. The foundation tool for all of Marcia's styling begins with her:
    C. *Blow-dryer*
        A blow-dryer is an electrical device designed for drying and styling hair in a single service. The blow-dryer is considered a basic necessity for today's stylist.

89. Marcia's blow-dryer must have a/an ____attachment that allows the hair to be dried as if it was being air dried.
    C. *Diffuser*
        A diffuser attachment causes the air to flow more softly, which in turn, allows the hair to dry so as to accentuate its natural texture and definition.

90. To detangle wet hair before blow-drying, Marcia will need to purchase a:
    C. *Wide-toothed comb*
        The wide-toothed comb allows the stylist to easily comb through the hair and prepare it for styling.

91. For her clients with mid- to longer length hair, Marcia will need a ____ .
    B. *Paddle brush*
    > The paddle brush has a large flat base, ball tip, and staggered nylon pins, and is great for use on mid- to long hair lengths because it does not snag or catch the hair.

92. For clients with fine hair or for adding lift at the scalp area, Marcia will need a:
    C. *Vent brush*
    > A vent brush has a ventilated design and is useful in speeding up the drying process, as well as for adding volume at the scalp area.

93. For clients who need a strong hold styling preparation, Marcia picks up:
    C. *Styling gel*
    > Styling gel is a thick, usually clear preparation, that has a strong hold factor and is used to create strong hold or control in styles.

94. For clients who want to add weight to their hair and achieve a piecy, textured look, Marcia purchases:
    D. *Styling pomade*
    > Styling pomade adds considerable weight to the hair by causing hair strands to join together and by causing significant separation in the hair.

95. To add gloss and shine to a finished style, Marcia will need:
    C. *Silicone shiners*
    > Silicone shiners are used to add shine and gloss to the hair without adding weight. These products may also create textural definition.

THERMAL HAIR STRAIGHTENING

96. In order for Shereen to style Ternyce's hair, she will need to determine:

    D. *How much curl to remove from it*

       Shereen will need to know what type of finished look Ternyce is trying to achieve, then assess the natural curl in her hair to best determine how much curl to remove and how to accomplish the style.

97. To remove 100 percent of Ternyce's curl, Shereen will need to use a:

    C. *Hard press*

       A hard press involves the application of the thermal pressing comb twice on each side of the hair to adequately remove all of the curl.

98. Before pressing, Shereen should add ____ to Ternyce's hair and scalp.

    C. *Pressing oil*

       Adding pressing oil will make the hair softer and prepare and condition it for the pressing treatment, as well as protect the hair and scalp from the heat of the comb.

99. To remove 100 percent of Ternyce's curl, and to then curl the hair around the face and under at the nape, Shereen will need to use a:

    D. *Double press*

       When double pressing, the stylist will first straighten the unwanted curl and then recurl the hair into the direction and amount of curl that is desired for the finished look.

Chapter 13

BRAIDING AND BRAID EXTENSIONS

CLIENT CONSULTATION, UNDERSTANDING THE BASICS, AND BRAIDING THE HAIR

100. Lolita explains that complicated braid styles can last for up to:
D. *90 days*

Since many braids are beautifully complex and can take several hours to complete, they can, if taken care of, last for as long as three months before they need to be rebraided or touched up.

101. One of the most important aspects of Lolita's client consultation will be to assess the _____ of Darshan's hair.
D. *Texture*

Darshan's hair texture—whether coarse, medium, or fine, whether oily, dry, or wiry, and whether straight, curly, or coiled—will all be very important clues as to what hairstyle will work best for him and be easy to maintain.

102. Lolita determines that Darshan would look best in a braid style that is full on top and at the neckline, but close to his head at the temples because she has determined that he is a/an _____ facial type.
D. *Diamond*

A diamond face shape is widest at the center of the face and requires that a hairstyle, in order to balance the face, adds fullness to the forehead and jawline areas.

103. In addition to the combs, brushes, and blow-dryer Lolita will need for the service, she also sets up her station to include the extension materials, ____, and ____.
C. *Drawing board and hackle*

A drawing board has flat leather pads and fine teeth that sandwich the human hair extensions and allow the needed hair to be extracted without disturbing or loosening the rest of the hair. A hackle is a board with fine nails used to detangle and comb out the hair.

104. Since Darshan intends to wash his hair every two weeks and let it dry naturally without the use of heat or irons, and he desires a shiny, reflective finished look, the material Lolita considers using is:
C. *Nylon*

Since nylon is a synthetic fiber that delivers high shine and can reflect light, and based on how Darshan plans on caring for his hair, it is the perfect choice for his extension material.

105. Darshan explains that he wants a braid that looks like two strands of hair wrapped around one another, called a/an:
B. *Rope braid*

The rope braid is made with two strands that are twisted around each other. This technique can be used on layered or one-length hair.

Chapter 14

WIGS AND HAIR ENHANCEMENTS

WIGS

106. For clients who want the highest quality wigs to cover 100 percent of their hair, Carlotta orders:

   C. *Human hair wigs*

   Human hair wigs are of the best quality and look the most natural because they react to wear just as natural hair would.

107. If a client is interested in a product that is ready-to-wear, that comes in fantasy colors, and whose color will not fade, Carlotta should recommend a:

   A. *Synthetic wig*

   Synthetic hair wigs can simulate natural hair wigs, are less expensive, are usually ready to wear and easy to care for, and can come in lots of interesting and attractive colors.

108. For a client who is interested in an airy type of wig that is less structured, Carlotta should suggest a:

   B. *Capless wig*

   A capless wig is one that is less structured and is open, airy, light, and comfortable to wear.

109. To measure a client for a wig, Carlotta will need a:

   C. *Soft tape measure*

   A soft tape measure is useful for measuring around the contours of the head.

110. When customizing the wig to the exact requirements of the client, Carlotta is best able to make alteration to the wig:

   B. *On a block*

   A block is a head-shaped form, usually made of canvas covered cork or foam to which the wig is secured for fitting, cleaning, coloring, and styling.

HAIR EXTENSIONS

111. Before attaching any hair extensions, Linda will need to ascertain from Judy whether or not to:
    B. *Add length to the overall style*
       Judy will need to decide how much length she wants to add to her existing hair.

112. When attaching an extension, it should be placed:
    D. *About one inch from the hairline*
       It is a general rule of thumb to stay about one inch from the hairline, in the front, at the temples, and at the part line when attaching extensions.

113. Since Judy has fine hair, Linda will need to:
    C. *Be careful to hide the base of the hair weft*
       Since fine hair is usually also thinner than coarse hair, it will be important for Linda to be aware of where she is attaching the weft of hair, and to be sure to have enough hair and length above it to cover the weft.

114. The best method Linda can use for attaching the hair weft to Linda's fine hair is the ____ method.
    D. *Fusion*
       In the fusion method, the extension hair is bonded to the client's own hair by a heat activated bonding material. This is best for fine hair because it doesn't leave any bulk to cover up when completed.

Chapter 15

CHEMICAL TEXTURE SERVICES

THE CLIENT CONSULTATION AND PERMANENT WAVING

115. Anna's hair texture indicates to Mark that her hair may:
C. *Require more processing time*
Based on her hair texture, Anna has coarse hair which usually requires more processing time.

116. Since Maureen's hair is colored, Mark must take special care to notice her hair's:
A. *Porosity*
Since Maureen's hair has been colored, she has already opened the cuticle layer of her hair and slightly damaged it, so Mark will need to assess how much damage the hair has undergone in order to asses the porosity level, the hair's ability to absorb liquid, and prepare accordingly.

117. When wrapping Anna's hair, Mark will employ the ____ technique in order to achieve a tighter curl at the ends and a looser curl at the scalp.
C. *Croquignole*
Using the croquignole means the hair is wrapped from the ends to the scalp in overlapping layers, which produce a larger curl at the scalp and a tighter curl at the ends.

118. In order to achieve uniform curl throughout the entire hair strand, Mark will wrap Reva's long hair using the ____ technique.
A. *Spiral*
Using the spiral wrap technique, the hair is wrapped either from the ends to the scalp or from the scalp to the ends, evenly and without much overlap, so the result is more even curl formation.

119. To achieve a tighter curl in the center of each strand and a looser curl on the outer edges, Mark will use ____ rods when wrapping Maureen's hair.
   B. *Concave*
      Concave rods have a smaller circumference in the center of the rod and a wider circumference on the outside edges, which produces a tighter curl on the inside of the curl.

120. To protect the many layers in Maureen's haircut while perming, Mark will employ the ____ wrap.
   B. *Double flat*
      The double flat wrap employs two end papers, one under the hair and one over the hair to protect the hair and its layers when wrapped around the rod.

121. To perm Anna's thick, coarse hair, Mark should select a/an ____ wave.
   A. *Exothermic*
      An exothermic wave has an alkaline pH of 9.0 to 9.6 and employs a heat reaction during the waving process.

122. To perm Maureen's extremely damaged hair, Mark should select a/an ____ wave:
   B. *True acid*
      A true acid wave with a pH of 4.5 to 7.0 is best used for extremely damaged hair or extremely porous hair, and is perfect for Maureen's hair.

123. To perm Reva's virgin hair, Mark should select a/an ____ wave:
   A. *Cold*
      A cold or alkaline wave, with a pH of 9.0 to 9.6, is perfect for hair that is coarse, thick, and resistant such as Reva's hair.

PERMANENT WAVE PROCESSING

124. Based on Mrs. Carr's description of her hair, her hair is:
C. *Overprocessed*
Overprocessed hair usually has a weak curl or results in straight hair.

125. The perm solution that Jill chose was most likely too:
C. *Strong*
Overprocessed hair means that the waving lotion was either too strong or left on the hair too long.

126. Mrs. Carr's hair doesn't have enough strength left to:
C. *Hold the desired curl*
Mrs. Carr's hair doesn't have the strength to hold the curl because too many disulfide bonds were broken during the perming process.

CHEMICAL HAIR RELAXERS AND EXTREMELY CURLY HAIR

127. To completely straighten Charlotte's hair, Margie will use a:
B. *Chemical hair relaxer*
Using a chemical hair relaxer is the only way to permanently remove all of the curl from Charlotte's hair to achieve her desired look.

128. To remove some of the curl from Barbara's hair, Margie will use a:
C. *Soft curl permanent*
Since Barbara only wants to have more control over the amount of curl she wears instead of eliminating it completely, Margie will use a soft curl permanent to reform the curl.

129. What should Margie do to determine Charlotte's reaction to the service?
D. *Use a protective base*
Since Margie knows that Charlotte has a sensitive scalp, she should opt to use a protective base to

protect her scalp before the application of the straightener.

130. A relaxer containing which of the following active ingredient is most appropriate for Margie to use on Charlotte's hair, given her sensitive scalp?
    D. *Guanidine hydroxide*
        Guanidine hydroxide has a pH of 13 to 13.5, causes less skin irritation than other hydroxide relaxers, and is a good choice for someone like Charlotte.

131. What strength relaxer is best used on Charlotte?
    A. *Mild*
        Since Charlotte's hair has already been colored, a mild formula is the best choice for a straightening product.

132. Barbara's soft curl perm will:
    C. *Reformulate the amount of curl she has*
        A soft curl perm does not remove curl; it simply changes the type and amount of curl so that it is easier to work with.

133. How many services are required for Margie to perform the soft curl perm on Barbara's hair?
    B. *2*
        A soft curl perm requires two services. The first is a relaxing service with a thio relaxer; the second is the wrapping of the relaxed hair on tools to reform the curl.

134. Which of the following is involved in Margie performing the soft curl perm on Barbara's hair?
    B. *Relaxing the hair and then recurling it*
        This process doesn't really straighten the hair; what it actually does is make the client's existing curl softer and looser.

Chapter 16
HAIRCOLORING

COLOR THEORY

135. To counteract the greenish tinge in Mary's haircolor, Danny will need to select a shade that has a ____ base color.
   C. Red
   > To counteract a greenish tinge to hair, Danny will need to determine which color is opposite the color he wants to cover on the color wheel and use a new shade to change the greenish hair to a more natural shade.

136. To prevent Mary's highlighted hair from becoming too dark during the correction procedure, Danny must be careful not to add too much ____ to the color formulation.
   A. Blue
   > The addition of blue to a color darkens the overall shade.

137. The color Danny will use to correct Mary's haircolor is a ____ color.
   A. Primary
   > A primary color is a pure or fundamental color that cannot be achieved through a mixture of other colors.

138. To return Amber's haircolor to the desired shade, Danny will need to use a ____ tone.
   D. Cool
   > Since Amber complains that her hair is too brassy or orangey (warm tones), Danny will need to use a cool shade to counter the red tones.

139. Typical colors in the tone range Danny will use on Amber's hair have a ____ base.

    D. *Blue*

    Any cool color will have some degree of blue in its base tone.

140. The color Danny will use to correct Amber's brassy tone is a/an ____ color.

    B. *Complementary*

    Complementary colors are a primary and a secondary color positioned opposite each other on the color wheel.

141. Once achieved, Amber's haircolor will be a level:

    D. *3*

    A level is a unit of measurement used to identify the lightness or darkness of a color. If Danny achieves the dark brown shade Amber desires, he will have achieved a level 3 hair color for her.

142. If Zeena wanted her bleached hair to have a cooler, more platinum look instead of the lemony color it is now, Danny will need to select a shade that has a ____ base.

    D. *Violet*

    To counteract the lemon yellow color, Danny would need to choose a blue-based color for Zeena. Violet is a blue-based color and is opposite yellow on the color wheel, making it the right choice for a platinum blond look.

143. If Zeena wanted her bleached hair to have a strawberry blond color instead of the lemony color it is now, Danny will need to select a shade that has a ____ base.

    C. *Red*

    A strawberry blond shade is a mixture of yellow and red, so since the hair is already very yellow, Danny would need to use a red-based shade on Zeena to achieve the strawberry color.

144. A strawberry blond shade would indicate that Zeena preferred a ____ tone in her hair.
    A. *Warm*
        Any color with a red or yellow base is a warm color.

145. Once achieved, Zeena's haircolor will be a level:
    A. *10*
        A level 10 is the lightest shade, and since Zeena wishes to be a platinum blond, she is asking for the lightest shade.

THE LEVEL SYSTEM AND TYPES OF HAIRCOLOR

146. Since Gina has about 25 percent gray, what is the overall situation Susan will encounter when coloring Gina's hair?
    C. *Gina has more pigmented hair than gray hair*
        Susan's assessment of Gina's hair is that she has 25 percent gray, which means that the remaining 75 percent of Gina's hair is pigmented.

147. To effectively blend Gina's gray hair, Susan should use a:
    C. *Demipermanent color*
        Demipermanent haircolor is a deposit only haircolor, which means that it does not lighten the hair during the coloring process. It deposits color and coats the hair shaft with dark color, which is an excellent way of coating and, therefore, blending gray hair with pigmented hair.

148. The type of color product Susan uses on Gina should:
    C. *Deposit color*
        Since the only required outcome of this service is to deposit color onto the unpigmented hair, the only thing the color needs to do is cover the gray.

149. When formulating Gina's color to ensure proper coverage, Susan should:
    D. *Select a shade two levels lighter than the desired shade*
        Since demipermanent color simply "dumps" color onto the hair shaft, it is important that the shade not become too dark to naturally blend with the

pigmented hair. It is usually recommended that a
lighter shade be used.

150. To achieve the chunky highlights that Maya desires,
Susan will need to use a/an:
D. *Off-the-scalp bleach*
Since chunky highlights appear in various areas on
the head and not at the scalp, an off-the-scalp bleach
is appropriate for use.

151. Since Maya's natural hair color is a bright shade of red-
orange, her hair will go through ____ degrees of
decolorization to achieve the yellow base shade she
desires for her highlights.
C. *5*
The darker the natural color of the hair, the more
stages of lightening the hair will go through. Since
Maya's hair is already a red-orange shade, she will
have to go through five more stages of decolorization
to achieve the blond highlights she requested.

152. Since Maya has so much red pigment in her hair
naturally, Susan may opt to use a ____ technique to
achieve a pleasing finished tone to the highlighted hair.
C. *Double process coloring*
A double process technique, which involves first
bleaching the hair and then toning it with a haircolor
shade, will help Susan get rid of the unflattering red-
orange tones that are naturally present in Maya's hair.

153. To lighten Katie's regrowth area, Susan will use a/an:
A. *On-the-scalp bleach*
Since the regrowth area is at the scalp, Susan will
need to use an on-the-scalp bleach to lighten Katie's
regrowth.

154. To boost the lifting power of the cream bleach, Susan will
use a/an:
B. *Activator*
An activator is an oxidizer added to hydrogen
peroxide to increase its chemical action, in this case,
its lifting power.

155. Before applying the toner to Katie's hair, Susan may choose to use a/an _____ to protect and condition the previously bleached hair.

    D. *Conditioner filler*

    A conditioner filler is used to recondition hair prior to the haircolor application. Color can be applied right over the conditioner filler and in this way, work together to color and condition the hair.

156. After her hair is lightened to the desired level, Susan should formulate and tone Katie's hair using a _____ volume developer to simply add color and lessen the amount of damage done to the hair.

    A. *10*

    Since the hair will have been lightened already, a low-volume developer is all that is needed for toning the prelightened hair.

157. Which of Susan's clients requires a patch test before she begins their services?

    D. *All of them*

    Since all of Susan's clients received color services using an aniline derivative tint, they all require a patch test.

Part IV   Skin Care

Chapter 17

HISTOLOGY OF THE SKIN

ANATOMY OF THE SKIN

1. During her examination, Donna is observing Clare's:
   A. *Epidermis*

   The epidermis is the outermost layer of the skin and provides the body with a thin protective covering.

2. Clare's tan is a result of the effect of ultraviolet rays that increased the amount of ____ in her skin.
   C. *Melanin*

   Melanin protects the sensitive cells below the skin from the destructive effects of the sun.

3. The appearance of skin that is taut, pink, and dry indicates that Clare may have a:
   C. *Sunburn*

   Skin that is taut, pink, and dry indicates that it has been overexposed to the damaging ultraviolet rays of the sun and that those rays have caused it to burn.

4. What is causing Clare's wrinkles?
   B. *Loss of collagen and elastin*

   Collagen is a fibrous protein that gives the skin form and strength. As the fibers become weakened, the skin begins to sag and wrinkle.

5. Which nerves are responsible for the pain Clare feels?
    B. *Sensory nerve fibers*
        Sensory nerve fibers are the ones that react to cold, heat, touch, pressure, and pain, and these receptors send messages to the brain.

6. Which nerves are responsible for Clare's nose being oily?
    D. *Secretory nerve fibers*
        Secretory nerve fibers are connected to the sweat and oil glands of the skin, and they regulate perspiration and the flow of sebum.

7. The nerves that are responsible for Clare's nose being oily are located in the _____ of the skin.
    C. *Reticular layer*
        The reticular layer is the deeper layer of the dermis that supplies the skin with oxygen and nutrients.

8. The dark spots that are imbedded in the skin on Clare's nose are called:
    B. *Comedones*
        A comedone is a worm-like mass of hardened sebum in a hair follicle.

9. These dark spots are caused by:
    A. *Hardened sebum in a hair follicle*
        These spots appear most frequently on the nose and forehead, and create a blockage at the mouth of the follicle.

10. These dark spots are considered to be a disorder of the:
    C. *Sebaceous glands*
        The sebaceous glands are connected to the hair follicles and they secrete sebum, a fatty or oily secretion that lubricates and preserves the softness of the hair.

DISORDERS OF THE SKIN

11. Gigi's perspiration is a function of the:
    C. *Sweat glands*
       The sweat glands regulate body temperature and
       excrete sweat from the skin. Sweat glands are more
       numerous on the palms, soles, forehead, and in the
       armpits.

12. The itchy, swollen lesion caused by Gigi's mosquito bite is
    called a:
    D. *Wheal*
       A wheal is an itchy, swollen lesion that lasts only a
       few hours and is caused by a blow, insect bite, or skin
       allergy.

13. While running, the sweat glands in Clare's ____ make
    adjustments to allow her to be cooled by the evaporation
    of sweat.
    B. *Skin*
       The skin protects the body from the environment
       and from overheating by making the necessary
       adjustments to allow the body to be cooled by the
       evaporation of sweat.

14. To protect herself from overexposure to the sun while
    running, Gigi should have worn a:
    C. *Sunscreen*
       Since overexposure to the sun can be damaging to
       the skin and can cause premature aging of the skin, it
       is best to always wear one and to advise clients to
       wear a sunscreen.

15. As a result of scratching the mosquito bites on her arms,
    Gigi had developed a/an:
    B. *Excoriation*
       An excoriation is a skin sore or abrasion caused by
       scratching or scraping.

16. The mass of small red bumps that burn when Gigi moves her arms back and forth are called:

    C. *Milaria rubra*

    Milaria rubra is an acute inflammatory disorder of the sweat glands, commonly known as prickly heat.

17. The foul odor Gigi notices after removing her running shoes is called:

    D. *Bromhidrosis*

    Bromhidrosis is foul-smelling perspiration, usually noticeable in the armpits and on the feet.

18. Brent's hands contain:

    C. *Calluses*

    Calluses are mounds of hardened skin that can accumulate on a person's hands or feet in areas that are frequently rubbed or to which friction is applied.

19. Pam's discolored spot is called a:

    A. *Stain*

    A stain is an abnormal brown or wine-colored skin discoloration with a circular or irregular shape.

20. What caused the discolored spot on Pam's forehead?

    C. *There is no known cause*

    The cause is unknown but stains have been discovered after long illnesses, during aging, and after the disappearance of moles.

21. Mrs. Fagan's outgrowths of skin are called:

    B. *Skin tags*

    A skin tag is a small brown or flesh-colored outgrowth of the skin that most frequently appears on the neck.

22. When do these outgrowths normally appear?

    B. *When a person ages*

    These skin tags normally appear when a person ages.

23. What is the dark colored spot on Maryanne's chest?
    C. *A mole*
       A mole is a small brownish spot or blemish on the skin that can range in color from a light tan to black. Large, dark hairs can also occur in moles.

CHAPTER 18

HAIR REMOVAL

CLIENT CONSULTATION, AND PERMANENT AND TEMPORARY METHODS OF HAIR REMOVAL

24. Before determining the appropriate methods of hair removal, a positive answer to which of the following questions would indicate to Amber that she should not be providing hair removal services for Joanie?
    C. *Do you currently use Retin-A?*
       The use of Retin-A or similar products is a contraindication for hair removal, which means that it should not be considered for use.

25. When Joanie shapes her own eyebrows with the pair of tweezers, she is using a method called:
    D. *Temporary hair removal*
       Tweezing is a form of temporary hair removal because the hair that is removed will grow back.

26. If Amber was to discuss methods of permanent hair removal with Joanie, she would suggest:
    D. *Electrolysis, photoepilation, and laser hair removal*
       Electrolysis is removal of hair by the use of an electric current, photoepilation is the removal of hair by means of an intense light to destroy hair follicles, and laser hair removal uses a laser beam pulsed on the skin to impair the hair follicles.

27. A quick and easy method of temporary hair removal Amber could suggest for removing the hair on Joanie's legs that would not leave the skin smooth but requires a patch test is:
    A. *A depilatory*
       A depilatory is a caustic substance that is applied to the areas and dissolves the superfluous hair at the skin level.

28. A milder but equally effective way of removing Joanie's facial hair could be to:

    D. *Sugar*

    Sugaring is an epilation treatment that employs a thick sugar-based paste and is especially appropriate for people who have sensitive skin.

29. To minimize the irritation to Joanie's underarms, Amber suggests the use of:

    D. *Cold wax*

    Cold wax is not heated before it is applied and is, therefore, milder for use on sensitive areas.

Chapter 19

FACIALS

BASIC CLASSIFICATION AND CHEMISTRY OF SKIN CARE PRODUCTS

30. Anne asks Rebecca about the difference between a face wash and a cleansing cream. Rebecca tells her that:
    D. *A face wash is a detergent-like foaming cleanser; a cleansing cream dissolves makeup quickly*
    A face wash is best used on a person with oily skin, while a cleansing cream is best used on a client with very dry or mature skin.

31. Jane explains that she has some acne and asks what she should use to cleanse her face. Rebecca suggests a:
    B. *Face wash*
    Using a face wash can cut excess amounts of oil on oily or combination skin.

32. For Andrea's dry and sensitive skin, Rebecca recommends using a/an ____ after cleansing.
    C. *Freshener*
    A freshener, which has the lowest percentage of alcohol, is beneficial for dry and mature skin as well as for sensitive skin conditions.

33. Jane complains that her skin appears bumpy and lumpy. Rebecca recommends that she use a/an ____ two to three times a week.
    D. *Exfoliant*
    An exfoliant is an ingredient that when added to a facial preparation, aids in the peeling and shedding of the horny outer layer of the skin.

34. Andrea tells Rebecca that her facialist suggested an enzyme peel but that she wasn't sure what it was. Rebecca responded by explaining that it is a/an:
    D. *Exfoliating procedure using keratolytic enzymes*
    > An enzyme peel is a chemical exfoliation whereby dead skin cells or the intercellular "glue" that holds them together is dissolved by a chemical agent.

35. Jane asks Rebecca if there is anything she can use on her skin daily to reduce dryness. Rebecca suggests a:
    C. *Moisturizer*
    > A moisturizer is a product formulated to add moisture to the skin.

36. Andrea wonders if there is any special treatment that can be useful on oily skin. Rebecca explains that a ____ mask will help reduce sebum production.
    C. *Sulfur*
    > Sulfur masks, which have sulfur as their main ingredient, have been found beneficial in reducing the production of sebum.

FACIAL MASSAGE

37. Alma begins by using a technique that involves a light, continuous, stroking movement called:
    B. *Effleurage*
    > Effleurage involves a light, continuous, stroking movement applied with the fingers or the palms in a slow, rhythmic manner; no pressure is used.

38. To offer deep stimulation to Patricia's muscles, Alma employs:
    A. *Petrissage*
    > Petrissage is a kneading movement performed by lifting, squeezing, and pressing the tissue with a light, firm pressure.

39. To increase Patricia's circulation and glandular activity, Alma uses a ____ technique.
 C. *Friction*
    Friction is a deep rubbing movement in which pressure is applied to the skin with the fingers or palms while moving over an underlying structure.

40. Alma uses ____ on Patricia's neck to tone her muscles.
 C. *Tapotement*
    Tapotement consists of short, quick, tapping, slapping, and hacking movements.

41. Alma is always careful to massage from the:
 C. *Insertion to the origin*
    Muscles that are massaged in the incorrect direction could result in the loss of resiliency and sagging of the skin and muscles.

ELECTROTHERAPY AND LIGHT THERAPY

42. Joyce asks if there is any electrotherapy treatment that will help liquefy sebum on the face of a client. Albert explains that the application of ____ will do just that.
 A. *Galvanic current*
    Galvanic current is the most commonly used and can produce significant chemical changes to the skin.

43. To tone the facial muscles of older clients, Joyce is interested in using:
 C. *Faradic current*
    Faradic current produces impulses on the muscles that force them to contract; it is a useful means of toning the muscles of aging clients.

44. For use on acne-prone skin, Albert explains the use of ____ will help the skin accept the treatment more deeply.
 D. *High-frequency current*
    High-frequency current has a germicidal effect, which makes it very useful for acne-prone skin.

45. To soothe Mark's aching back, Paulette will place him under a/an ____ light.
    B. *Infrared*
    Infrared light heats and relaxes the skin, and its deep penetration relieves pain in sore muscles and soothes the nerves.

46. To reduce Michelle's skin eruptions, Paulette will place her under a/an ____ light.
    A. *Blue*
    Blue light produces some chemical and germicidal effects, and can be used for mild cases of skin eruptions.

47. To alleviate Allie's sore shoulders and neck, Paulette will place her under a/an ____ light.
    C. *White*
    White light is used to relieve pain in the back of the neck and shoulders.

48. Amy will tan under a/an ____ light.
    D. *Ultraviolet*
    Ultraviolet light improves the flow of blood and lymph, and produces a tan.

49. To reduce the appearance of Mrs. Halperin's dry and wrinkled skin, Paulette will use a ____ light.
    A. *Red*
    Red light penetrates the deepest and improves dry, scaly, wrinkled skin.

Chapter 20

FACIAL MAKEUP

COSMETICS FOR FACIAL MAKEUP

50. From the information that Sandra has received about Amanda's color preferences and from analyzing her skin, she determines that her skin tone is:

    D. *Warm*

    A warm skin tone is evident if the client has yellow undertones in her skin and looks best in gold, red, or orange shades.

51. Before any other product goes on Amanda's face, and to even out her skin tone and create a base for the makeup application, Sandra uses:

    B. *Foundation*

    Foundation is a tinted cosmetic that is used as a base or as a protective film before makeup or powder are applied.

52. To cover Amanda's blemish and to reduce the discoloration around her eyes, Sandra will apply a concealer whose color is:

    B. *The same as the skin tone*

    A concealer that is matched to the skin color is best to blend in skin blemishes and discolorations.

53. To set the foundation, concealer, and to give the face a matte finish, Sandra pats on a:

    C. *Face powder*

    A face powder is a fine cosmetic powder used to add a dull or matte finish to the face.

54. To keep her makeup matte looking natural, Sandra adds _____ cheek color.

   C. *Dry*

   Dry cheek color imparts a matte finish and is applied with a brush or cotton puff.

55. To harmonize with Amanda's coloring, she should wear a _____ color on her cheeks.

   C. *Coral*

   A coral shade will harmonize with Amanda's red hair and her warm skin tone.

56. To keep Amanda's lip color from feathering, Sandra applies:

   D. *Lip liner*

   Lip liner is a colored pencil used to outline the lips prior to the application of lipstick.

57. Sandra fills in Amanda's lips with:

   A. *Lip color*

   Lip color is applied to enhance the natural color and shape of the lip or to redefine the lip. Lip color is available in a myriad of shades and glosses.

58. The best lip color to apply is:

   A. *Warm toned*

   A warm toned color will have orange and red undertones, and is best for use with a makeup palette of similar tones.

59. To make Amanda's green eyes a focal point, Sandra should select a _____ color.

   C. *Plum*

   Since red is the color opposite green on the color wheel, a red-toned color will be best to accentuate green eyes.

60. Sandra highlights Amanda's eyes with a color that is:

   A. *Lighter than the skin tone*

   Highlighting is a technique used to draw attention to a certain area; in this case, a color lighter than the natural skin tone will draw attention to the eyes.

61. To make Amanda's eyes appear larger and more open, Sandra should apply:
    D. *Mascara on top and bottom lashes*
       Curling the upper lashes and applying mascara to both the top and bottom lashes will make the eyes appear larger and more open.

CORRECTIVE MAKEUP

62. What face shape does Courtney have?
    D. *Inverted triangle*
       Courtney has a face shape that is wider at the forehead and narrower at the chin. This is called an inverted triangle.

63. To make Courtney's face appear more oval, Linda will need to:
    B. *Minimize the width of the forehead and increase the width of the jawline*
       To achieve the most desirable look for her client, Linda will want to reduce the appearance of the forehead while making the jaw appear wider.

64. To make Courtney's small eyes appear larger, Linda will:
    D. *Extend the eye shadow above, beyond, and below the eyes*
       To make small eyes appear bigger, Linda will extend the eye shadow around the eyes, making them look larger than they actually are.

65. To create more fullness to Courtney's neck and jawline area, Linda decides to apply a ____ to the area.
    C. *Light foundation*
       Since light colors attract attention, and since Linda wants to make the neck area appear larger, she will use a light color foundation in this area.

66. To make Carmen's round face appear slimmer, she will need to:
    D. *Slenderize and lengthen the face*

    Linda will use a darker foundation around the outside perimeter of Carmen's face to make her face seem slimmer and more oval-shaped.

67. To correct Carmen's wide, flat nose, Linda will:
    C. *Apply a dark foundation on either side of the nostrils*

    By applying a dark foundation on either side of the nostrils, Linda will reduce the appearance of the nose width.

68. To minimize her protruding eyes, Carmen should:
    B. *Blend a deep shade of shadow over the upper lid and to the eyebrow*

    A medium to deep eye shadow shade should be used over the prominent part of the upper lid, carrying it lightly toward the eyebrow.

69. To slenderize Carmen's neck and jawline area, Linda will apply a ____ to the area.
    A. *Dark foundation*

    A dark colored foundation will make a wide neck and jaw area appear slimmer.

70. To give the appearance of a more balanced face, Rita can offset her low forehead with eyebrows that have a:
    C. *Low arch*

    A low arch gives more height to a very low forehead, resulting in a balanced look to the face overall.

71. How can Linda correct Rita's thin upper lip?
    C. *By using a lip pencil to make the curves of the upper lips proportionate to the nostrils*

    To increase the size and appearance of her thin upper lip, Linda can use a lip pencil to draw in the peaks of the upper lips, using the nostrils as a guide, and then filling in the lip with a medium to light colored lipstick.

Part V   Nail Care

Chapter 21

NAIL STRUCTURE AND GROWTH

NAIL GROWTH AND NAIL DISORDERS

1. While recovering from a serious heart attack, Mrs. Jones'
    nails developed wavy ridges. Ellie recognized the condi-
    tion as:
    B. *Corrugations*
        Corrugations or wavy ridges are caused by the
        uneven growth of the nails, usually the result of
        illness or injury.

2. Ruben gave his daughter a gift certificate for a manicure
    with Ellie in the hopes that it would arrest her
    onychophagy, a condition where she ____ her nails.
    C. *Bites*
        Nail-biting is the result of an acquired nervous
        habit that prompts the individual to chew the nail or
        the hardened cuticle around the nail.

3. After losing more than 100 pounds on a fad diet, Sabrina
    noticed that her nails were noticeably thinner, whiter,
    and more flexible than normal. Ellie explained that this is
    called ____ .
    B. *Eggshell nails*
        Eggshell nails have a noticeably thin, white nail
        plate and are more flexible than a normal nail. The
        nail usually separates from the nail bed and curves
        around the free edge.

4. Raul has very thick nails that seem to grow in layers. He has:

   C. *Onychauxis*

   Onychauxis is an overgrowth of the nail, usually in thickness rather than in length, and may be caused by a local infection, internal imbalance, or heredity.

5. After Sabrina slammed her hand into the table when she fell at home, she noticed a whitish discoloration of her nails. Ellie told her this was called ____ and caused by injury to the base of the nail.

   C. *Leukonchia*

   Leukonchia are white spots that appear on the nail after injury to the base of the nail bed, but do not necessarily indicate disease of the nail.

6. What is the green spot?

   B. *A bacterial infection*

   This discoloration is a bacterial infection caused by a naturally occurring bacteria on the skin that has grown out of control. Under the correct circumstances, it causes an infection.

7. The green spot is most likely caused by:

   B. *Trapped moisture between the natural nail and the enhancement*

   Infection can be caused by the use of contaminated implements or by moisture that has been trapped between an unsanitized natural nail and an artificial nail enhancement such as a tip or wrap.

8. How will this nail most likely be cured?

   C. *By exposing it to air*

   Since this bacteria is an anaerobic bacteria, it cannot live in the presence of oxygen, so by removing the artificial nail enhancement and exposing the area to the air, the bacteria will die.

NAIL DISEASES

9. The first slide Dr. Reddy shows is of a nail that is separated from and falling off of the nail bed. This condition is called:

    C. *Onchomadesis*

    > Onchomadesis is usually caused by a local infection, minor injuries to the nail bed, or severe systemic illness.

10. The next slide depicts a nail with an inflamed matrix with pus and shedding. This condition is called:

    A. *Onychia*

    > Onychia can occur from any opening of the skin that will allow bacteria, fungi, or foreign materials to enter.

11. Dr. Reddy shows another slide and explains that growth of horny epithelium in the nail bed is called:

    D. *Onchophosis*

    > Onchophosis refers to the growth of horny epithelial in the nail bed.

12. Dr. Reddy's next slide is of a man's foot with what appear to be deep, itchy, colorless blisters. These are:

    A. *Athlete's foot*

    > Athlete's foot or tinea pedis appears as isolated blisters or in groups on both or only one foot, and can spread over the sole and between the toes of the feet.

Chapter 22

MANICURING AND PEDICURING

NAIL CARE TOOLS

13. The first thing that Josie does is:
    C. *Remove the old nail polish*
    Before she does anything else, Josie must remove Wanda's old nail polish so that she can clearly see the nails and fingers.

14. To shape Wanda's nails, Josie will use a/an:
    D. *Emery board*
    An emery board is a disposable manicuring implement with two abrasive sides used for shaping and smoothing the nail.

15. Wanda explains that she would like her nails shorter, so Josie uses a ____ to shorten them to the desired length.
    D. *Nail clipper*
    A nail clipper is a reusable metal instrument used to shorten very long nails.

16. Josie recommends that Wanda consider using a ____ daily to correct and prevent brittle nails and dry cuticles.
    C. *Cuticle cream*
    A cuticle cream, designed to prevent or correct brittle nails and dry cuticles, is safe to use every day.

17. Before applying the polish and base coat, Josie applies a ____ to strengthen the nails and prevent them from splitting or peeling.
    D. *Nail hardener*
    Nail hardeners or strengtheners are designed to prevent nails from splitting or peeling, and are applied to the nail before the base coat.

18. How should Josie remove excess nail polish from around Wanda's nails?
    B. *With a cotton-tipped orangewood stick dipped in polish remover*
       Josie will carefully wipe a cotton-tipped orangewood stick dipped in polish remover over the areas where the excess polish appears and clean up her polish lines.

PEDICURES

19. Before getting to the foot massage, Joya must:
    B. *Clip and file toenails, file down rough skin, and place the feet in the foot bath*
       Before a professional nail technician begins a foot massage, she will want to have evaluated and cleaned the client's foot and prepared it for the massage.

20. To push back the cuticle and finish the pedicure, Joya will use a:
    D. *Cuticle solvent and a cotton-tipped orangewood stick*
       Joya will use a cuticle remover that is a solution of alkali, glycerin, and water to soften and remove dead cuticle from around the nail.

21. Once the pedicure is completed, Joya will begin the massage with the ____ technique for relaxation.
    C. *Effleurage*
       The effleurage technique is a light or hard stroking movement, employed on top of the foot.

22. Next, Joya will move on to a ____ massage technique, which will promote flexibility and stimulate blood flow.
    D. *Metatarsal scissors*
       The metatarsal scissors technique is a petrissage or kneading movement that promotes flexibility and stimulates blood flow.

23. To further stimulate blood flow, Joya will use the _____ technique.
    C. *Fist twist*
       This movement allows the hand to be twisted on the bottom of the client's foot and used to help stimulate blood flow.

24. Joya will end the massage with a technique called _____ to reduce the blood flow.
    B. *Percussion*
       The percussion technique involves a light tapping over the entire foot to reduce blood circulation at the end of the service.

DISINFECTING FOOT SPAS

(Please refer to Chapter 5, Infection Control, page 115, in *Milady's Standard Cosmetology*, 2004 ed.)

25. Heather instructs Allie to _____ after draining the water and removing foreign matter from the foot spa after each client.
    B. *Clean the surfaces and walls with soap and water*
       The foot bath must be cleaned with soap or detergent after each client, then rinsed with clean, clear water.

26. Next, Heather explains that Allie will need to disinfect the foot bath with a/an _____ disinfectant, according to the manufacturers' directions.
    C. *EPA-registered*
       All foot baths and/or spas must be disinfected with an EPA-registered disinfectant that has bactericidal, fungicidal, and viricidal efficacy.

27. At the end of each day, Heather tells Allie that she will need to:
    D. *Remove the screen and clean the debris trapped behind it*
       At the end of the day, Allie will need to remove the screen from each foot bath that has been used, clean out the debris that will have collected there as a result

of performing pedicure services, and wash the screen and inlet with a soap or detergent and chlorine solution.

28. When washing the screen and inlet, Allie may use a ____ percent chlorine solution.
    A. 5

    A 5 percent chlorine solution, which can be made by mixing 5 percent chlorine bleach to one gallon of water, may be used to disinfect the foot spa instead of washing the spa and then totally immersing in an EPA-registered disinfectant.

29. To flush the system at the end of the day, Allie should use a low-sudsing soap and warm water, and allow it to filter through the system for:
    C. 10 minutes

    Flushing the system for 10 minutes at the end of the day with soap and water is recommended. Then Allie should rinse, drain, and allow the foot spa to air dry.

30. Heather tells Allie that every two weeks she will need to fill the foot spa tub with water and four teaspoons of 5 percent bleach solution and let the solution sit:
    C. Overnight

    This solution should sit in the foot spa tub overnight. Then in the morning, before customers come in for service, the tub should be drained and the system should be flushed with clear, clean water.

Chapter 23

ADVANCED NAIL TECHNIQUES

NAIL WRAPS

31. In order to determine the best type of wrap for Kelly, Roberta will need to ask her which of the following questions?
    C. *How rough are you on your hands and nails?*
       Each type of nail wrap has specific elements that make it more suitable for one type of client over another. By asking Kelly how she uses her hands, Roberta will be in the best position to recommend a suitable procedure for her needs.

32. Kelly explains that she is a landscape artist, and she works outdoors planning and gardening all day long. Based on this, Roberta recommends that she wear _____wraps for durability.
    C. *Linen*
       Linen provides a durable wrap and is much thicker than silk or fiberglass. Linen requires a colored polish to cover the material once applied.

33. Kelly asks Roberta about maintaining her new nails. Roberta explains that her nails must be:
    B. *Glued every two weeks and rewrapped every four weeks*
       Proper maintenance of linen wrapped nails ensures that the nails stay healthy and look good.

34. Joanne wears nail tips with acrylic overlays, so when Roberta does Joanne's nails, she uses:
    B. *A monomer and polymer*
       Acrylic nails require the use of monomer (a clear liquid) and a polymer (a white powder) to be applied to the nail and dried.

35. To aid in the adhesion and to prepare the nail surface for attachment with the acrylic material, Roberta will use ____ on Joanne's' nails.
    D. *Primer*
    A primer is a substance that improves adhesion and prepares the nail surface for bonding with acrylic material.

36. Once applied, acrylic overlays should be ____ every two weeks and the shape of the nail should be ____ each time acrylic is used.
    D. *Filled, balanced*
    Every two weeks, additional acrylic must be applied to the nail growth. This is called a fill. In addition, because more acrylic material is being applied to the nail, the nail will need to be smoothed out or balanced to accommodate the new acrylic.

37. The completion of Nicole's gel nail application will require Roberta to use two steps: ____ and ____ .
    C. *Application, hardening*
    The gel nail wrap is in liquid form and is applied with a brush. Once applied, it will need to be cured or hardened.

38. Roberta chooses a no-light gel for Nicole's nails, so she may need to ____ to finish the nail application.
    C. *Immerse Nicole's hands into water*
    The act of immersing the hand with the gel overlay on it into the water will harden the gel substance so that the rest of the service can be completed.

Part VI The Business of Cosmetology

Chapter 24

THE SALON BUSINESS

GOING INTO BUSINESS FOR YOURSELF

1. Emily tells Don that she is a ____ , which means that she pays rent to a salon owner for the space she works in, supplies all of her own materials and products, and has complete control over her work schedule and appointments.

   C. *Booth renter*
   > Booth renting is a very popular way of becoming your own boss, especially for someone who wants flexibility but not the responsibility of managing others.

2. Scott is a ____ of the Scott Salon and is responsible for determining all the policies of the salon, hiring and paying all the employees, and he assumes all the responsibilities of the expenses and profits of the salon.

   D. *Sole proprietor*
   > A sole proprietorship is a situation where one person, the owner of the business, has all of the responsibilities and reaps all of the rewards.

3. Matt explains that he is a ____ with his wife, Anne. They share all of the duties of owning the business and all of the rewards as well. Since he is a cosmetologist, he manages the salon while his wife, who is an accountant, manages the finances and operations.
   A. *Partner*
      In a partnership, two or more people own the business together. Usually, these individuals bring different, complementary skills to the partnership.

4. Scott advises Don to be aware of the area in which he will be working. He explains that ____, ____, ____, and ____ are important factors in determining where to open a new salon and whether or not it will be successful.
   B. *Demographics, visibility, parking, competition*
      It will be important for Don to know who his clients are, where they will and won't go, and how best to position his salon over the other salons that will compete for the same type of clients.

5. Don's friends advise him to develop a ____, which will help him clarify his vision and determine which type of opportunity is best for him.
   B. *Business plan*
      A business plan is a document that forces the entrepreneur to thoroughly think through all of the aspects of his business and make decisions up front so that he has a clear vision.

6. John asks Don how much ____ he is seeking to run the salon for the first two years.
   C. *Capital*
      Capital refers to the amount of financial support, or money, will be needed to run the business for the first two years of operation.

7. John asks Don what percentage of the overall salon revenue he expects to spend on rent for the space and for advertising.
   C. *Approximately 16%*
      Typically, space rental for a business such as a salon should be about 13 percent of the gross income and

advertising should comprise about 3 percent of the gross income for a total of 16 percent.

8. To make informed decisions about the salon's financial success, Don explains to John that he will keep ____ and ____ records to control expenses and waste.
   D. *Weekly, monthly*
      Weekly and monthly records allow the salon owner to make comparisons from one year to the next, detect changes in demands for goods and services, check on the use of materials, and control expenses.

9. Don mentions that ____ supplies such as hairspray and styling products will be on hand to sell to salon clients so that they can maintain their styles at home, and that these sales will increase the salon's profitability.
   D. *Retail*
      Retail supplies are those products that are on hand for the sole purpose of reselling them to salon clients.

10. John asks to see a copy of the projected ____ so that he can assess whether or not the salon will have the correct flow, and be conducive to the many services and the demands of the clients who will patronize it.
    C. *Salon layout*
       A salon layout is a drawing or plan that assesses the flow of traffic and people through the space, and allows the new owner to determine if the space is used efficiently and wisely.

OPERATING A SUCCESSFUL SALON AND MANAGING PERSONNEL

11. As the salon manager, and to help his staff ease into the move, Andrew should:
    B. *Be honest about the situation and provide updates when they are available*
       Being honest with salon staff is the only way for Andrew to ready them for the upcoming changes, and to keep an atmosphere of honesty and trust with his staff.

12. Since Andrew knows that once the move is announced, some of his longtime staffers may experience feelings of uncertainty and fear, he offers to:

C. *Listen and help them with their issues*

   Andrew's responsibility is to be a caring and professional salon manager. Helping or advising his staff to take their clients and go to another salon would be unethical, but he can offer to listen to the staff's feelings and try his best to help solve any concerns they may have.

13. For those decisions that he can share with his staff, and for those issues that can be resolved by the staff, Andrew should consider:

B. *Sharing the decision-making with the staff when it is feasible to do so*

   Allowing the staff to take part in some of the decision-making, when it is feasible to do so, will enlist them in the overall decision and calm their fears of being powerless in the situation.

THE FRONT DESK

14. Marta should:

C. *Excuse herself briefly from the client and answer the call*

   While she wants the client in front of her to feel valued and important, Marta also has a responsibility to answer the telephone promptly. If she politely asks the client to excuse her for a moment to answer the call, she attends to both clients' needs perfectly.

15. If Marta chooses to answer the call and help the caller, how should she resume her conversation with the upset client?

B. *By determining when the stylist can begin her service and offering to reschedule her appointment if she prefers*

   Marta must be prepared to do whatever she can to make the client happy, fix her problem, and accommodate her schedule. Rescheduling at the client's convenience is a good approach.

16. If Marta chooses not to answer the call, she may be missing an important opportunity for the salon to:
    B. *Change an appointment for a client*
       Marta really doesn't have the option of not answering the call. Whether someone is calling to make or change an appointment, Marta is paid to answer the phone and help clients. The salon is dependent on her ability to do so flawlessly.

17. To make the upset client happy and to keep her as a salon regular, Marta should:
    D. *Ask how she would like to remedy the problem and get approval from salon management*
       Marta can simply ask the client what she prefers and how she would like the issue to be resolved, thus ensuring that the client gets the kind of satisfaction she desires. Once she ascertains this information from the client, Marta should speak with and get the approval of her salon manager before proceeding.

Chapter 25

SEEKING EMPLOYMENT

PREPARING FOR LICENSURE AND THE TEST, AND DEDUCTIVE REASONING

18. Samuel should begin studying:
    D. *Several weeks before the exam*
       By giving himself several weeks to study for something as important as the state board exam, Samuel has plenty of time to review all of his subjects and to concentrate on topics that are not quite clear to him instead of cramming a few days before the exam.

19. In order to get ready for his written exam, Samuel should:
    D. *Review past quizzes, tests, and homework assignments*
       Using his past homework assignments, tests, and quizzes is an excellent way to prepare for the exam as they are sure to cover the most important pieces of data and remind him of vital information he may have overlooked.

20. The evening before the exam, Samuel should plan to:
    D. *Get a full night's sleep*
       The best thing Samuel can do the night before the exam is to get enough rest and sleep to ensure that he feels great in the morning, is calm, well prepared, and clear-thinking for the exam.

21. Once he is given the exam, Samuel should:
    C. *Read through the exam and all of the directions before beginning the test*
       It is always best to read through all of the information on a test before plunging into answering the questions, although that may have been Samuel's first reaction. This gives the test-taker an overview of the test and of what is expected.

22. If Samuel is stuck on a question, he can ____ and then determine which are possible correct answers.
    B. *Eliminate answers he knows are incorrect*
       Since all of the state board written exams are multiple choice format, Samuel can go through the possible answers and eliminate those that he knows are incorrect. This will leave him with one or two that are most appropriate. He can asses the possibilities from there.

PREPARING FOR EMPLOYMENT

23. When she arrives at the first salon, the manager asks Amira for her credentials. She should hand her a:
    B. *Resume*
       A resume is a written summary of education and work experience, and it is expected that a person applying for a job would have one.

24. What kinds of information will the manager need to ascertain about Amira before determining if she is right for the open position?
    B. *Her job history*
       The manager will want to know what type of jobs Amira has held, how much responsibility she was entrusted with, and for how long she remained in each position.

25. Another tool Amira should consider taking with her on interviews is a/an:
    C. *Employment portfolio showing before and after photos of past clients*
       Creating a portfolio of styles that she has created will help the salon manager determine the caliber of Amira's work and determine what additional training or practice she may need once hired.

26. In order to validate her claim that she has been a responsible employee while working for others, Amira should provide:

C. *Letters of reference from past employers*

Letters of reference will tell Amira's new manager exactly how she will perform and what she can expect from others who have managed Amira in previous employment.

27. After having met and spent some time with the salon manager, Amira should send:

D. *A "thank-you" note for the interview*

It is considered both polite and professional to thank an interviewer for the time and energy she spent interviewing you for a position with her firm or salon.

28. If she is offered the position, Amira will have to decide ____ before taking the job.

C. *If the salon has the kind of image, culture, and values that she has*

It is always important for a new employee like Amira to really understand the salon's image, culture, and values, and feel like their beliefs match her own. Otherwise, Amira could be setting herself up for failure.

Chapter 26

ON THE JOB

OUT IN THE REAL WORLD

29. Sara tells Marshall that the salon operates very much like a/an ____ in that everyone is aware of his own duties but is also ready and must be willing to aid coworkers in whatever needs to be accomplished.

    B. *Team*

    A team environment is an excellent environment for a salon. In a team situation, every person has value and knows how his work affects the overall salon. And each person also knows that the team leader, or salon manager, is available for help or assistance if needed.

30. Sara explains that payday is on Friday and that he will make a ____, which is a percentage of his service dollars and an hourly wage.

    D. *Salary plus commission*

    Salary plus commission is an excellent way for a new stylist to get paid when he is beginning at a new salon because he is guaranteed a salary and is also rewarded with a commission on his service and retail dollars.

31. Sara explains that after his first 90 days of employment, Marshall will have a/an ____, which will be an opportunity for her to assess his progress and performance and for Marshall to discuss his thoughts and ideas about the salon.

    B. *Employee evaluation*

    An employee evaluation is an excellent way to determine and define expectations, both for Marshal's expectations of the salon and for the salon's expectations of Marshall.

32. Marshall asks Sara if she can help him determine what his paychecks might be for the first three months of employment so that he can make a ____ to track his expenses such as loan repayments and household expenses.
    C. *Personal budget*
    A personal budget is an invaluable tool for every salon stylist to have whether new to the business or a 20-year veteran. A personal budget will enable Marshall to know where he sits financially every month and help him make financial decisions responsibly.

33. Sara assigns Marshall to Joyce, a senior stylist, who will be responsible for answering his questions, giving him guidance, and helping him when he has difficulty. Joyce will be his:
    D. *Mentor*
    Having a senior stylist as a mentor is a tremendous asset for Marshall because she will be someone who can help him, answer his questions, and give him individual guidance and attention whenever he needs assistance. Joyce's only intention will be Marshall's complete and successful transition into this new salon life.

DISCOVER THE SELLING YOU

34. When Noreen comes in for her haircut and styling appointment, Sheniqwa should:
    D. *Review Noreen's record card and discuss the condition of her hair*
    For a client such as Noreen, even weekly shampooing and styling can add undue burden on her fragile hair, so Sheniqwa is right to review her record card and her hair condition each time she comes into the salon so that she can make appropriate recommendations.

35. While discussing her hair, Noreen mentions that she is having difficulty with her hair being so dry and looking so dull. Sheniqwa will want to use this as an opportunity to:

    A. *Discuss the new line of retail products to Noreen and how they can benefit her*

        By listening to Noreen, Sheniqwa gets lots of clues as to what her client needs and what she can provide in terms of solutions, whether additional services or products.

36. Since Noreen's hair is very dry and damaged, Sheniqwa suggests adding a deep conditioning treatment to today's service. This is called:

    B. *Ticket upgrading*

        A ticket upgrade is the practice of recommending and selling additional services to clients that may be performed by yourself or someone else in the salon.

37. Once Noreen has had her service and sees the benefit of the treatment, Sheniqwa can use a ____ approach to recommending additional retail products for at-home use.

    C. *Soft sell*

        A soft sell approach is one in which Sheniqwa can easily suggest that Noreen purchase the product or service because Noreen herself has either already requested it or has benefited from it.

38. In order to obtain important demographic information on her clients, Cassie will need to refer to her:

    B. *Client record cards*

        The client record cards, if filled in properly, should contain the demographic information Cassie needs such as addresses, birth dates, and how often they frequent the salon.

39. Cassie notes that she can use her business cards to:

    B. *Promote a referral program with current clients*

        A referral program using business cards is the most logical and the easiest of all of the referral programs a stylist can use. Cassie will simply give her business card to current clients, ask them to write their names on the card, and pass them along to their friends. Once the card is received by Cassie, the person whose name appears on it gets an additional discount on their next service.

40. As a reward for her loyal clients, and to promote the purchase of additional services and products, Cassie can prepare a ____ and include it in a "thank-you" or birthday card mailing.

    C. *Discount coupon*

    Taking a small 10, 15, or 20 percent discount on regular services or products is a great incentive and "thank you" for loyal clients.

41. To make herself visible to new groups of potential clients, Cassie could:

    C. *Make herself available to speak at local organizations*

    By offering her time to speak at local organizations and groups, Cassie becomes visible and positions herself as an authority in the area of beauty and grooming, which encourages people to take part in her service offerings.

42. Cassie could make use of her relationships with other local merchants by:

    B. *Agreeing to cross-promote with merchants who are willing to do so*

    Cross-promoting with other businesses such as florists, bakeries, and drycleaners is an excellent way to advertise services to other business' clients that do not compete with your business.

43. Cassie realizes that one of the simplest ways to increase her business is to:

    B. *Listen to clues clients give and offer services to accommodate their needs*

    Most of the time, her clients come into the salon with needs Cassie can handle if she is willing to listen to what her clients are saying and then provide them with the solutions they need.

Index

Page numbers for **Answers** are in **bold**